MRI from A to Z

Second Edition

Gary Liney

MRI from A to Z

A Definitive Guide
for Medical Professionals

Second Edition

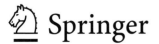 Springer

Author
Gary Liney, PhD
Principal Physicist
Oncology Imaging
and Radiotherapy Physics
Queen's Centre for Oncology
Castle Hill Hospital
Cottingham
UK

ISBN: 978-1-84996-134-9   e-ISBN: 978-1-84996-135-6

DOI: 10.1007/978-1-84996-135-6

Springer Dordrecht Heidelberg London New York

A catalogue record for this book is available from the British Library

Library of Congress Control Number: 2010930086

Cover design: eStudio Calamar Figueres/Berlin

Printed on acid-free paper

Springer is part of Springer Science+Business Media (www.springer.com)

For DJ, Becks and Matty Man

Preface

The long-awaited second edition is ready. So what has happened in the last 5 years? Quite a lot by the look of it! Parallel imaging is now commonplace whereas it only merited a fleeting mention in the first edition. Numerous clinical high-field systems have been installed, which continue to drive the applications forward. Techniques such as hyperpolarization are knocking loudly on the door of the clinician. Contrast agents have expanded beyond recognition. MRI continues to find new areas of utility and is increasingly used in combination with other medical imaging modalities. The distinction between research and clinical practice has become ever more blurred with all the MRI vendors continuing to deliver exciting new products on the cutting-edge. The vocabulary needed to keep up with all of this has increased exponentially, and of course there are even more pulse sequence acronyms to puzzle over. This is all reflected in the text which is almost 80% bigger than the first edition and thanks to Springer there are also a lot more figures in this one too. Every entry has been re-appraised and updated where necessary. In total there are now over 1,300 entries (according to my daughter who patiently sat and counted them!). It has been quite a toil keeping up with it all but I hope you find it useful.

Gary Liney
Cottingham, UK

Acknowledgments

All images were acquired in Hull, East Riding of Yorkshire, England.

Thanks to The Centre for MR Investigations, Hull Royal Infirmary and also the following individuals: Dave Manton, Rebecca Liney, Pete Gibbs, Roberto Garcia-Alvarez, Tim Jones, Sharon Burton, Chris Bilton, Shelley Waugh, Victor Lazar, and Richard Dunnington.

A

AB systems

Referring to molecules which exhibit multiple MRS peaks due to spin-spin interactions. In a so-called AB system, the *chemical shift* between each spin is of similar magnitude to the splitting constant (J). A common example is *citrate* (abundant in the normal prostate) which consists of two pairs of strongly coupled methylene protons (denoted A and B) such that: $v_A - v_B = 0.5J$ where v_A, v_B are the resonating frequencies of the two protons. A tall central doublet is split into two smaller peaks either side, which are not usually resolved in vivo at 1.5 T. Citrate exhibits strong *echo modulation*.

See also *J-coupling* and *AX systems*.

References

Mulkern RB, Bowers JL. Density matrix calculations of AB spectra from multipulse sequences: quantum mechanics meets spectroscopy. Concepts Magn Reson. 1994;6:1–23

Absolute peak area quantification

MR Spectroscopy method of obtaining metabolic concentrations from *peak area ratios* where the denominator is the water signal. The areas are adjusted for differences in relaxation times, and the actual concentration of the metabolite is determined from:

$$[m] = [w] \times \frac{2}{n} \times \frac{S_0^m}{S_0^w}$$

G. Liney, *MRI from A to Z*,
DOI: 10.1007/978-1-84996-135-6_1,
© Springer-Verlag London Limited 2010

where [w] is the concentration of water and S_0 are the peak area amplitudes of the metabolite and water signals at equilibrium i.e., having been corrected for the relaxation, which has occurred at the time of measurement. The factor 2/n corrects for the number of protons contributing to the signal (here 2 is for two protons on the water molecule). The concentration of water is taken as 55.55 mol kg^{-1}.

References

Barker PB, Soher BJ, Blackband SJ, Chatham JC, Mathews VP, Bryan RN. Quantitation of proton NMR spectra of the human brain using tissue water as an internal concentration reference. NMR Biomed. 1993;6:89–94

Acoustic damping

Description of a method for reducing the *acoustic noise* of the scanner by using gradient coils that have a suitable insulating material such as foam or rubber inserted between the inner coil and outer shielding coil.

Acoustic noise

The audible noise produced by the scanner when in operation. Specifically, it is due to vibrations in the gradient coils caused by the Lorentz Force. This is induced by the rapidly oscillating currents passing through the coils in the presence of the main magnetic field. Ear protection must by worn by patients because of this noise. Gradient intensive sequences, e.g., 3D GRE, EPI etc produce the highest noise levels. Reported noise levels are often weighted (on the so called dB (A) scale) to account for the frequency response of the human ear. Values of 120 dB (A) have been recorded with EPI sequences. The *Lorentz force*, and therefore noise level, increases with field strength (typically a 6 dB increase from

1.5 to 3.0 T). Current methods to combat noise include mounting the gradient coils to the floor to reduce vibrations and mounting them within a vacuum and/or use of *acoustic damping* material. More sophisticated measures include *active noise reduction*.

See also *bore liner* and *vacuum bore*.

References

Shellock FG, Ziarati M, Atkinson D, Chen DY. Determination of gradient magnetic field-induced acoustic noise associated with the use of echoplanar and 3D fast spin-echo techniques. J Magn Reson Imaging. 1998;8:1154

Acoustic shielding

Referring to the reduction of *acoustic noise* transmitted from the scan room itself by insulating the walls with appropriate materials.

Acquisition time

Time taken to acquire an MR image. For a spin-echo sequence it is given by:

$$N_p \times N_A \times TR$$

where N_p is the number of *phase encoding* steps, N_A is the number of signal *averages*, and TR is the *repetition time*. Reducing any of these terms shortens scan times with the following trade-offs in image quality of spatial resolution (N_p), signal-to-noise ratio (*SNR*) (N_A) and contrast (TR). Scan times may also be reduced by using *parallel imaging*.

In gradient-echo sequences with very short TR times, the above equation includes a factor for the number of slices acquired.

Activation map

A colored *overlay* that demonstrates the areas of brain function in an *fMRI* scan. It is produced by the pixel-by-pixel
calculation of *correlation coefficient* which compares the signal intensity changes with the timing of the experiment (see
paradigm). Pixel values that exceed a user-defined threshold
are highlighted and overlaid onto the grayscale images usually a separate high resolution data set for anatomical location. An example activation map is shown in Fig. 32.

Active noise reduction

An advanced method of reducing the gradient noise produced from the scanner. It utilizes force-balanced coils, which
are designed so that the *Lorentz Force* acts in a symmetrical
manner to counteract the vibrations. The method offers up to
30 dB reduction in noise.

See also *acoustic noise*.

References

Bowtell RW, Mansfield PM. Quiet transverse gradient coils: Lorentz
force balancing designs using geometric similitude, Magn Reson
Med. 1995;34:494

Active shielding

Refers to either shielding of the main magnetic field or the
gradient coils. The *fringe field* may be actively shielded using
an additional set of coil windings around the main set, with
a current of opposite polarity passing through it. Without
shielding the *footprint* of the scanner would be unacceptable.
As an example, an unshielded 7.0 T scanner has a five gauss
fringe field of 23 m.

See also *five gauss line* and *passive shielding*.

Gradients can be similarly shielded and are now standard on all systems. This reduces *eddy currents* in the *cryostat* and the other conducting structures.

Active shimming

The action of improving the homogeneity of the main magnetic field (the *shim*) by passing current through additional sets of coils within the scanner to augment the field. This is particularly important in MR spectroscopy. Typically 12 to 18 sets of coils are used which affect the field in each orthogonal direction. A first order shim changes the field in a linear fashion, a second order shim produces field changes that vary with the square of distance and so on (so called higher order shims). The shim coils themselves may be resistive or superconducting.

See also B_0 *inhomogeneity* and *passive shimming*.

ADC

1. Abbreviation for the Apparent Diffusion Coefficient. Refers to the measurable value of diffusion rather than the actual value due to the effects of cell boundaries etc. The signal attenuation observed in a Diffusion-weighted image (see *DWI*) due to the apparent diffusion coefficient, D, is:

$$S = S_0 . \exp(-bD)$$

where b is the gradient factor (see *b-factor*).
The ADC value for water is approximately $2.1 \times 10^{-3} \, \text{mm}^2 \text{s}^{-1}$.

References

Issa B. In vivo measurement of the apparent diffusion coefficient in normal and malignant prostatic tissues using echo-planar imaging. JMRI. 2002;16:196–200
See also *exponential ADC*.

2. ADC is the abbreviation for Analog-to-Digital converter, which digitizes the measured MR signal before further processing.

ADC map

A specific *parameter map* in which the pixel intensity is equal to the value of apparent diffusion coefficient (*ADC*). The map may be obtained from images acquired at several different values of *b-factor*. Care must be taken in selecting a minimum b value as flow effects dominate at very low b. Alternatively a two-point method may be used typically acquiring a b=0 image and a second image at a higher b value. ADC maps do not provide any directional information on their own but have found use in the early detection of stroke (see *DWI*) (Fig. 1).
   See also *DTI*.

Adenosine

See *stress-perfusion agent*.

Adenosine triphosphate

See *ATP*.

Adiabatic pulse

Specific use of a variable frequency *excitation pulse* which is swept through the Larmor frequency. These pulses are less sensitive to B_1 inhomogeneities than conventional pulses but take longer to apply. Used in *continuous wave NMR*.

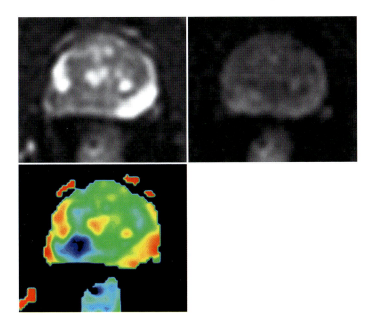

FIGURE I Images taken from a diffusion study in the prostate. The first two images are EPI scans with b-factors equal to 0 (*left*) and b=700 s mm⁻² (*right*). The resulting *ADC map* (*bottom*) demonstrates reduced values (*blue*) in the area of tumor. Liney G. MRI in clinical practice. London: Springer; 2006, p. 95

Agarose gel

A jelly-like substance derived from seaweed which may be used in the construction of phantoms. Its T_2 *relaxivity* (10 mM⁻¹ s⁻¹) is much higher than corresponding values for T_1 (0.05 mM⁻¹ s⁻¹). This means T_2 values can be made to vary considerably with little alteration in T_1. The material is often mixed with *Gd-DTPA* to produce phantoms with a range of T_1 and T_2 values in order to test the accuracy of relaxation time measurements.

See also *gel phantoms* and *gelatin*.

References

Mitchell MD, Kundell HL, Zxel L Joseph PM. Agarose as a tissue equivalent phantom material for NMR imaging. Magn Reson Imaging. 1986;4:263–266

AIF

Abbreviation for Arterial Input Function. This is the signal-time characteristic of the contrast agent bolus in the blood, and may be used to model uptake in other tissues. For best results an artery near to the site of interest needs to be selected for the appropriate AIF. This function is then deconvolved from tissue or tumor enhancement in order to quantitate perfusion.

See also *dynamic contrast enhancement* and *perfusion imaging*.

Alanine

A brain metabolite observed in proton spectroscopy with a resonance at 1.48 ppm. It is often seen to increase in meningiomas (Fig. 2).

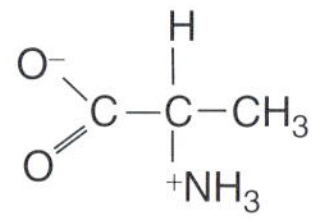

FIGURE 2 The chemical structure of *alanine*

Aliasing

Referring generally to image artifacts whereby anatomy is incorrectly mis-mapped onto the opposite side of the image. It occurs in the phase direction when anatomy extends beyond the imaging field of view but is still within the *sensitive volume* of the *RF coil*. It is seldom a problem in the frequency direction due to *oversampling*, which is always turned on with most MR scanners. The artifact is often avoided by preferentially swapping phase and frequency encoding directions. Aliasing is also referred to as wrap or foldover. An example is shown in Fig. 69.

See also *no phase wrap*, *frequency wrap* and *nyquist frequency*.

Alignment

Referring to the direction of the *net magnetization* vector when it is parallel to B_0 i.e., the situation prior to the first *excitation pulse*.

Alpha

Greek letter (α) used to denote *flip angle*.

Analogue-to-digital converter

See *ADC*.

Angiogenesis

A phenomenon typical of tumors where new blood vessel growth is induced (mediated by angiogenic factors) to meet the increased oxygen demand required for rapid development. This is utilized in *contrast enhanced* scanning in cancer, where there is a preferential uptake of the contrast agent by tumors, which improves its differentiation from surrounding normal tissue.

AngioMARK

Former commercial name of a *blood-pool agent* now known as *Vasovist*.

Angular frequency

A measure of the rotation rate. It is measured in *radians* per second with units of s^{-1} and is a multiple of normal *frequency*.

Anisotropy

A property of diffusion which is not the same in each direction i.e., it is non *isotropic*. Usually implies some preferred diffusion direction and can be used to elucidate structural information e.g., white matter fiber tracts in the brain.

See also *tensor*, *tractography*, and *fractional anisotropy*.

Anisotropy also describes spatial resolution, which is not the same in each direction e.g., in 2D imaging where slice thickness is often much greater than the in-plane resolution (anisotropic pixels).

Anterior

Referring to the front side of the patient anatomy. It is at the top of an axial image and on the left of a sagittal image (see Figs. 3 and 82).

See also *posterior*.

Antialiasing

See *no phase wrap*.

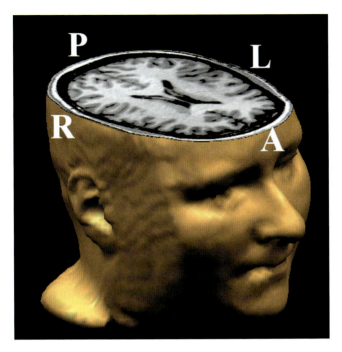

FIGURE 3 A 3D reconstruction of a brain volume which has been sliced in the *axial* plane. The image is labeled to indicate the anterior, posterior, left and right directions

Antiperistalsis

See *peristaltic motion.*

Apodization

An essential step in the post-processing of MR spectroscopy data. It involves the multiplication of the *free induction decay* signal by an appropriate filter to improve signal-to-noise and reduce truncation artifacts in the final spectrum. Filters include *exponential, Lorentzian* (a more rounded shape) and *Gaussian* (bell shaped). Filters may typically have a *linewidth* of between 2 and 4 Hz and their use results in a broadening of the spectral peaks.

Apodisation is also applied in the spatial domain to reduce voxel-voxel contamination (so called *voxel bleeding*) in MRSI. A common filter used for this is the *Fermi-filter*.

Apparent diffusion coefficient

See *ADC*.

ARC

Parallel imaging method from GE that stands for Auto-calibrating Reconstruction for *Cartesian* sampling. A self-calibrated technique similar to *GRAPPA* but with improved efficiency and reconstruction accuracy.

Area under the curve

The summation (integral) of the values in a series of sequential data points. A common example is in *dynamic contrast enhancement* where the area under the curve (also known as the positive enhancement integral) is a measure of the degree of contrast uptake. In certain cases (e.g., *perfusion imaging*) the effect and therefore the resulting area is a negative value.

Area under the curve (or AUC) is also used as a measurement of a receiver operating characteristic curve (see *ROC curve*).

Array

A combination of more than one RF *surface coil* to improve imaging coverage, taking advantage of the superior signal-to-noise of surface coils without the compromise of poor sensitivity of a single element.

In a *phased array* design, consideration of the overlapping profiles has to be taken into account. Phased array coils, like surface coils, are typically used as receive only coils (using the *body coil* to transmit). Coil arrays are now important in *parallel imaging* techniques.

Arrhythmia rejection

Technique used in cardiac gating whereby data is rejected if the *RR interval* exceeds a certain tolerance. This can lead to problems if the patient's heartbeat is irregular.

See also *trigger window*.

Artifact

Referring to any undesired signal contribution to the final image, which is not present in the real object or patient. Examples of common MR-related artifacts include *ringing, phase wrap*, *susceptibility artifact*, *chemical shift artifact* and *ghosting*. Various artifacts may be distinguished by their appearance and the encoding direction in which they propagate.

Arterial input function

See *AIF*.

Arterial spin labeling

A type of *perfusion imaging* method which does not require a contrast agent. Often abbreviated to ASL and sometimes further categorized as continuous (CASL) or pulsed (PASL). The technique works by acquiring a control image and a second image where the spins upstream are magnetically labeled in some manner so that they do not contribute to the final signal. These images can then be subtracted to produce an image that is based on perfusion. Several methods exist each employing different labeling and control approaches. Examples include *FAIR*, *EPISTAR* and *QUIPS*.

Artificial neural networks

Computational models, which mimic aspects of brain function and are used to classify or solve problems. Typically a data set is used to "train" the model and then it is "tested" on unseen data. They are designated as either supervised or unsupervised depending on the degree of user input at the training stage. They have been used in MRI for characterizing tissue types and tumor enhancement.

ASL

Abbreviation for *Arterial Spin Labeling*.

ASPIRE

GE sequence and acronym for Adiabatic SPectral Inversion Recovery Enhancement. A breast sequence using a longer than normal RF fat suppression pulse which is insensitive to B_1 *inhomogeneity*.

See also *adiabatic pulse*.

ASSET

Acronym for Array SenSitive Encoding Technique. The GE version of their *parallel imaging* method utilizing image based reconstruction.

Association fibers

Type of *white matter fibers* that connect different parts of the brain within the same hemisphere.

AST

Annotation on a *DICOM* image meaning *ASSET*.

Asymmetric echo

See *partial echo*.

Asymmetric sampling

Acquiring a reduced number of data points on one side of the *k-space* origin as a method of speeding up imaging time.
    See *partial k-space*.

ATP

Abbreviation for Adenosine TriPhosphate. Important compound observed in Phosphorus spectroscopy relating to energy. It consists of three spectral peaks referred to as α, β, and γ, with corresponding chemical shifts of -8, -15 and -4 ppm respectively. A phosphorus spectrum in shown in Fig. 70.

Attack

Referring to the initial slope of the gradient waveform from zero to its maximum amplitude, during the *rise time*. The equivalent *fall time* is sometimes referred to as the gradient decay.

AUC

Abbreviation for *Area Under the Curve*.

Auto shim

One part of the scanner *pre-scan* routine. Currents in the *shim* coils are adjusted until the maximum *homogeneity* in the imaging volume is achieved. A figure for the final *linewidth* of the water peak is usually provided as an indication of the success of the shim.

In imaging, auto shim is usually sufficient, whereas the stringent homogeneity required for MRS means that *manual shimming* is often additionally necessary.

See also *active shimming*.

Averaging

Improving the signal-to-noise ratio (*SNR*) by repeating the same part of a pulse sequence more than once. This works on the principle that signal is coherent whereas noise is random and its effect can be reduced by taking multiple measurements.

Increasing the number of signal averages proportionally extends the *acquisition time*, but with only a square root improvement in SNR.

See also *NEX*.

AVM

Abbreviation for Arterio-venous malformation.

AX systems

Molecules, which exhibit splitting of MRS resonances and where the chemical shift between the peaks is much greater than the coupling or splitting constant (J). Examples include hexachloropropane. AX systems also demonstrate weak *echo modulation*.

See also *J-coupling* and *AB systems*.

Axial

A 2D imaging plane taken in cross-section, dividing the subject into superior and inferior portions. *Slice selection* in this case is along the z-axis and the image is in the xy plane i.e., perpendicular to B_0.

Sometimes referred to as transaxial or transverse (Fig. 3).

See also *coronal*, *sagittal*, and *oblique*.

B

b-Factor

Term relating to the degree of sensitivity of a diffusion weighted sequence determined by its diffusion gradient characteristics. It is related to both the gradient amplitude and timing and for a typical *Stejskal-Tanner* bipolar sequence it is given by:

$$b = \gamma^2 \, G^2 \, \delta^2 \, (\Delta - \delta / 3)$$

where G is the diffusion gradient amplitude, δ is the gradient duration, and Δ is the interval between the trailing-to-leading edges of the two gradient pulses. Typical values of δ and Δ are between 30 and 40 ms. The $(\Delta-\delta/3)$ term is the *diffusion time*.

The above equation may be further modified to account for the *rise time* of these gradients. There will also be a small diffusion contribution from the normal imaging gradients which is not shown in this equation.

Images at different b-values can be acquired to characterize the apparent diffusion coefficient or *ADC* (usually $0 < b < 1,000 \, \mathrm{s\,mm^{-2}}$) (Fig. 4).

See also *DWI* and *diffusion time*.

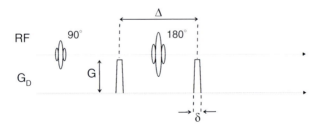

FIGURE 4 The gradient arrangement in a spin-echo diffusion-weighted sequence illustrating the gradient amplitude (G), the duration (δ) and the interval (Δ) which determine the *b-factor*

B$_0$

Conventional notation used to refer to the main or static magnetic field produced by the scanner. The direction of the main field is usually assigned the z-direction. Typical clinical scanners operate at 1.5 T but there are increasing numbers of *high field* systems.

Theoretically, the signal-to-noise ratio (*SNR*) increases as B$_0^{3/2}$, but due to changes in relaxation times, principally T$_1$, the actual relationship is nearly linear. (For example from 1.5 to 3.0 T the increase should be a factor of 2.8 but it is nearer 2.0).

See also *B$_0$ inhomogeneity*.

B$_0$ correction

Use of the water resonance in MRS to provide a chemical shift reference for the assignment of other metabolites, whose frequencies may alter across voxels due to B$_0$ inhomogeneity.

B$_0$ inhomogeneity

Changes in the main magnetic field due to either inherent manufacturing limitations or the introduction of some material into the scanner. The magnetic field becomes less homogenous the further away from the scanner *isocenter* and causes *geometric distortion*. This is particularly evident at the edges of large field-of-view images. Homogeneity is characterized by the *DSV* of the system and is best with a *superconducting magnet* but poorer for other magnet types or more open configurations.

See also *open scanner*.

B$_1$

Notation for the time-varying magnetic field produced by the *RF coil*, which is applied to excite and refocus spins etc. Its direction must be perpendicular to B$_0$ and applied at the

Larmor frequency. By convention the orientation of this field is in the xy plane (see *x-direction*). Typical values are of the order of 0.01 mT.

See also *RF power* and *flip angle*.

B_1 inhomogeneity

Changes in the RF field leading to artificial signal variation in the final image. The main contribution is from the B_1 profile of the receiver coil and the effect is most prominent with a *surface coil*. At high field strengths, conductive and dielectric effects cause additional inhomogeneities (see B_1 *doming*).

See also *coil uniformity correction*.

B_1 doming

Term used to describe the inhomogeneity observed in images at high field (3.0 T and above) due to the increased *dielectric effect*, which produces a *standing wave artifact*. The result is an increased signal at the center of the image. The effect can be especially prominent in phantom images and limits the maximum useful diameter of the test object. B_1 doming is accentuated by poor *RF penetration* leading to lower signal at the periphery. *RF shimming* may be used to improve uniformity across the image.

See also *wavelength*.

B_1 profile

The sensitivity of an RF coil to magnetic field (in the case of a receiver coil) or the variation in field strength produced as a function of distance from the coil (for a transmitter). Surface coils have characteristically poor reception profiles leading to marked B_1 *inhomogenity*.

See also *parallel imaging* and *coil uniformity correction*.

Balanced echo

See *bFFE*.

Banding artifacts

Bands of high signal appearing in steady state type sequences due to resonant offset effects. Methods of reducing these bands include averaging the effects (see *ROAST*) and using *rewinding gradients*.

Bandwidth

The frequency range of the *receiver*. It is related to the frequency used to encode each individual pixel and therefore determine the extent of the *chemical-shift artifact*. For example, using a 256 frequency encoding matrix and bandwidth of 32 kHz there is 125 Hz per pixel (=32,000/256) so the fat-water shift is approximately two pixels at 1.5 T. Typical bandwidths (BW) vary from 6.5 kHz to 1 MHz. Note that on GE scanners the bandwidth is given as ± half the full frequency range.

See also *variable bandwidth*.

Bandwidth per pixel

Sequence setting for adjusting the receiver bandwidth on Siemens scanners. It is equal to the receiver bandwidth divided by the imaging matrix in the frequency encoding direction.

See also *chemical shift artifact* and *variable bandwidth*.

Baseline

Referring to a signal intensity level or an image acquired under some reference condition e.g., a pre-contrast image prior to contrast enhancement or a resting state in some *fMRI* experiment. A stable signal baseline is a pre-requisite of any fMRI study (see *stability*).

In MRS it refers to the background noise level in a spectrum measured in a region away from the peaks of interest.

Baseline correction

The method of processing MR spectra which flattens the baseline signal making peaks easier to interpret. Usually needed to remove broad spectral humps which are exhibited by immobile macromolecules with short T_2^* values, which produce an elevation of the spectral baseline.

See also *rolling baseline*.

BASG

Acronym for BAlanced *SARGE*.

BEAT

Name given to the dedicated cardiac imaging system from Siemens.

See also *cardiac MRI*.

bFFE

Abbreviation for Balanced Fast Field Echo. A Siemens/Philips sequence, which may be described as a "True" FISP sequence i.e., it uses balanced *re-winding gradients* in all three directions to reset the phase at the end of each *TR*.

See also *FISP*.

Bind

Process by which images from two separate series are appended to produce a new image series. Also called concatenation.

Binomial pulse

A commonly used type of composite RF pulse where the individual flip angles are the coefficients of a binomial series (for example in multiples of 1:–1, or 1:–2:1 like *PROSET*). These are often used to suppress fat signal due to the dephasing of water and fat in between the sub-pulses (Fig. 5).

Bioeffects

Referring to any biological effects on the human body caused by the interaction with the MR scanner. These effects can be categorized into (1) static field (B_0) effects, (2) time varying field (*gradient*) and (3) radio-frequency (B_1) effects.

There are no known long-term or irreversible effects from exposure to fields below 10.0 T. Some studies have shown short term "mating-avoidance" in small mammals at 3.5 T. The biggest risk is from the *projectile* effect of ferromagnetic objects brought into the scan room.

The rapidly varying gradient fields have the potential to cause *peripheral nerve stimulation*. The most apparent effect of these however is *acoustic noise*.

Excessive radio-frequency interaction in patients will lead to tissue heating (see *RF heating*) with the possibility of *RF burns*.

See also *safety limits*.

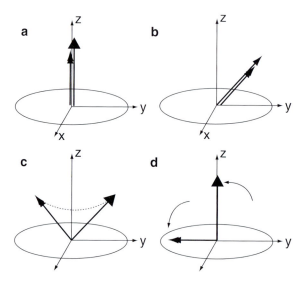

FIGURE 5 Example of a simple 1:–1 *binomial pulse*. In this example the first RF pulse tips both the fat and water 45° (**a, b**). The signals precess until they are out of phase (**c**) and then a second –45° pulse is applied (**d**). The water and fat are now separated so that either one can be imaged. In similar way a 1:–2:1 pulse can be used (with angles 22.5° and 45°). Liney G. MRI in clinical practice. London: Springer; 2006, p. 10.

Biot-Savart law

The law of physics that determines the magnetic field at a point due to a distribution of electrical currents.

The magnetic field (B) at a point R from a long straight wire carrying a current I, can be shown to be:

$$B = \frac{\mu_0 I}{2\pi R}$$

where μ_0 is the *permeability* of free space.

For a current loop of diameter a, the field a distance x away from its axis is:

$$B = \frac{\mu_0 I 2\pi a^2}{4\pi \left(x^2 + a^2\right)^{3/2}}$$

The field is maximum at the center of the loop (x = 0) and decreases further away. For distances $x \gg a$ this approximates to:

$$B = \frac{\mu_0 I a^2}{2\left(x^3\right)}$$

References

Gettys WE, Keller FJ, Skove MJ. Physics: classical and modern. New York: McGraw-Hill; 1989. ISBN: 007100453X

Bipolar

Used to describe a pair of gradients of equal amplitude but opposite direction in order to sensitize the imaging sequence to motion.

See also *Stejskal-Tanner*.

BI-RADS

Acronym for Breast Imaging Reporting And Data System. This is a standard diagnostic lexicon originally established for use in conventional mammography by the American College of Radiology, and now extended for MRI. A common set of reporting terms are used to describe things like morphological shape and enhancement kinetics of breast lesions (see *Type I,II,III…*).

See also *morphological descriptors.*
http://www.acr.org/

Birdcage

A very efficient *RF coil* design utilizing many regularly spaced conductors giving it its characteristic appearance and name (see Fig. 46). Sometimes referred to as a distributed capacitance coil, it consists of two circular conductive loops (known as end rings) connected by a number of straight segments (legs).

Most head and integrated body coils are of this design and typically used as a *transceiver*. These coils produce very homogenous imaging, particularly in the *axial* plane.

See also *saddle coil*, *solenoid* and *surface coil*.

References

Hayes CE, Edelstein WA, Schenck JF, Mueller OM, Eash M. An efficient, highly homogeneous radiofrequency coil for whole-body NMR imaging at 1.5 T. J Magn Reson. 1985;63:622–628

Bit

Smallest digital data unit (with a value equal to either 1 or 0). The term is an acronym of binary digit. One *byte* is made up of 8 bits. Image data (i.e., pixel intensity values) are typically stored as unsigned integers in 8 or (more usually) 16 bits.

Black blood

Referring to MR Angiography techniques in which blood (flowing spins) appears dark compared to stationary tissue.

See also *high velocity signal loss* and *white blood*.

BLADE

Siemens version of their motion correction technique using radial k-space acquisitions. It can be selected as a *k-space trajectory* option (instead of *cartesian*) and applied to any image sequence.

See also *PROPELLER*.

Bland-Altman plot

A comparison of two measurements to establish whether or not they are in agreement, for example two MR parameters. It is a plot of the difference against the mean of the two measures.

Blipped EPI

A common implementation of the EPI sequence in which the phase encoding gradient is applied by the same amount while the frequency gradient is switched from positive to negative in order to sample k-space in a regular trajectory (see Fig. 27).

Other methods include *spiral EPI* and *constant EPI*.

BLISS

A bilateral breast imaging sequence from Philips.

See also *VIBRANT*.

Bloch equations

The set of empirical equations first introduced by Felix Bloch in 1946 to describe the behavior of nuclear spin in a magnetic field under the influence of RF pulses.

The basis of the Bloch equations is the rate of change of net magnetization $\underline{M}$ when placed in an external magnetic field $\underline{B}$ which is given by:

$$\frac{d\underline{M}(t)}{dt} = \underline{M}(t) \times \gamma \underline{B}(t)$$

This was modified to account for the observed relaxation effects (T_1 and T_2) and can be simplified by adopting the *rotating frame* of reference. Under the conditions of free precession following a 90° pulse the equations become:

$$\frac{dM_z(t)}{dt} = \left(M_0 - M_z(t)\right)/T_1$$

$$\frac{dM_x(t)}{dt} = \gamma B_0 M_y(t) - M_x(t)/T_2$$

$$\frac{dM_y(t)}{dt} = -\gamma B_0 M_x(t) - M_y(t)/T_2$$

The solutions are as follows (where $\omega_0 = -\gamma B_0$):

$$M_z(t) = M_0(1 - e^{-t/T1})$$

$$M_x(t) = M_0 e^{-t/T2} \cos \omega_0 t$$

$$M_y(t) = M_0 e^{-t/T2} \sin \omega_0 t$$

This describes the familiar situation of the magnetization relaxing along the z-axis at the rate of $1/T_1$, while precessing in the xy plane (at a frequency ω_0) and relaxing at the rate $1/T_2$.

References

Bloch F. Nuclear induction. Phys Rev. 1946;70:460–473

Bloembergen, Purcell, and Pound equation

The equation, which relates tissue *relaxation* times to molecular tumbling rates and field strength. The motion of molecules can be represented by the *correlation time* or the time interval between collisions (of the order of 10^{-12} s). This will be influenced by structure and temperature, and in turn affects relaxation times. For effective T_1 relaxation the tumbling rate must be close to the *Larmor frequency*. In the extreme cases of either free water (e.g., CSF) or bound water, there are relatively few molecules at this rate and T_1 relaxation is long. In terms of T_2, slow moving molecules such as *bound protons* (e.g., proteins) experience net changes in local field variations and have short values but as tumbling rates increase these effects average out and longer T_2 values persist. Generally, tissue relaxation times will be a weighted average of free and bound components. The equations are shown below for completeness:

$$\frac{1}{T_1} = C\left[\frac{\tau_c}{1+\omega_0^2\tau_c^2}+\frac{4\tau_c}{1+4\omega_0^2\tau_c^2}\right]$$

$$\frac{1}{T_2} = \frac{C}{2}\left[3\tau_c+\frac{5\tau_c}{1+\omega_0^2\tau_c^2}+\frac{2\tau_c}{1+4\omega_0^2\tau_c^2}\right]$$

where τ_c is rotational correlation time, C is a constant dependent on *dipole-dipole interactions* and is ω_0 the resonant frequency.

The T_2 equation contains a zero-frequency component, which demonstrates the weak field strength dependence of T_2. In contrast, T_1 values become longer as field strength increases, as the proportion of spins tumbling at the resonant frequency is reduced.

See also T_1 and T_2.

Blood pool agent

Type of experimental *contrast agent* with a long vascular half-life so that it remains in the blood much longer than conventional contrast agents, which enter extravascular space due to their small molecular size. This has advantages for *contrast-enhanced MRA*. Many of the agents e.g., *AngioMARK*, bind reversibly to albumin.

References

Saeed M, Wendland MF, Higgins CB. Blood pool agents for cardiovascular imaging. J Magn Reson Imaging. 2000;12:890–898

Blood suppressed preparation

Referring to a pulse sequence which nulls the signal from blood thereby creating a *black-blood* image. It works by using a double inversion pulse, the first non-selective, while the second pulse re-inverts the slice thereby leaving it unchanged. The sequence is then timed so that blood flowing into the slice has reached the *null point* at the time of signal detection.

Blooming ball artifact

The large circular signal void caused by a *susceptibility artifact* and especially seen at the end of biopsy needles when the needle trajectory is along the direction of B_0.

See also *MR compatible*.

References

Lewin JS, Duerk JL, Jain VR, Petersilge CA, Chao CP, Haaga JR. Needle localization in MR-guided biopsy and aspiration: effects of field strength, sequence design and magnetic field orientation. AJR Am J Roentgenol. 1996;166:9

Blurring

The effect of reduced spatial resolution when using excessively long echo trains in *FSE* type sequences. It is caused by the increased discrepancy between the weighting of the individual signal echoes used and the overall *effective TE*.

Body coil

The RF coil which is usually integrated into the bore of the scanner and cannot be seen. Primarily used for body imaging where a large field-of-view (typically up to 40 cm) can be used. It is normally operated as a *transceiver*, and often of *birdcage* design.

BodySURF

Method of performing *whole-body screening* whereby the patient is moved on a board through a fixed RF surface coil arrangement to permit full coverage of the body. A specific whole-body MRA implementation of this technique has been referred to as AngioSURF.

Body vision

Toshiba's whole body diffusion imaging application.
    See also *DWIBS*.

Boil-off

Relating to the rate at which the *cryogen*s need replenishing to maintain the *critical temperature* of the *superconducting magnet*. Typical values are between 0.03 and 0.075 $L\,h^{-1}$ while some newer magnets have an effectively zero boil-off.

BOLD

Acronym for Blood Oxygen Level Dependent contrast. A specific type of *fMRI* technique, which monitors the haemodynamic response to brain activation. The increased oxygen fraction in the blood caused by local neuronal activation reduces the *paramagnetic* effect of deoxyhaemoglobin. This causes a small signal increase on T_2 or T_2^* weighted images of a few percent with the latter being most sensitive.
    The response lags the neuronal firing, by several seconds (see *haemodynamic lag*). Often the signal is characterized by an

initial dip as the increased demand for oxygen uses up the local supply before being replenished. There is also typically a characteristic overshoot in the activation and sometimes an accompanying undershoot at the end of the stimulus. This is thought to be mediated by a slow reacting change in blood volume.

References

Ogawa S, Lee TM, Nayak AS, Glynn P. Oxygen-sensitive contrast in magnetic resonance imaging of rodent brain at high fields. Magn Reson Med. 1990;14:68–78

Boltzmann constant

Physical constant equal to 1.381×10^{-23} J K^{-1} and used in the *Boltzmann distribution* equation.

Boltzmann distribution

The population distribution of spins between the *spin up* and *spin down* state. At room temperature and at clinical field strengths the tiny majority in the ground state (spin up) is of the order of 10^{-6} (i.e., one in a million).

The ratio of the spins in the two states at temperature T, is given by:

$$n_\beta / n_\alpha = \exp\left(-\Delta E / \kappa T\right)$$

where n_α and n_β are the number of spins in the spin-down and spin-up state respectively, ΔE is the energy difference between these states and κ is the *Boltzmann constant*.

The difference in populations can be approximated to:

$$n_\beta - n_\alpha \cong n\Delta E / 2\kappa T$$

where n is the total number of spins. The energy difference, ΔE is equal to $\hbar \gamma B_0$ where γ is the *gyromagnetic ratio,* $\hbar$ is the reduced *Planck's constant* and B_0 is the magnetic field. This means that increasing the field strength increases the population difference leading to a larger MR signal.

Bolus

Referring to the intravenous dose of a *contrast agent*. It may be performed by hand or preferentially by an automatic injector, triggered from the scanner control room, to deliver a reproducible delivery.

See also *AIF* and *transit time*.

Bolus timing

The synchronization between the arrival of the contrast agent at the site of interest (given by the mean *transit time*) and the acquisition of the imaging sequence. More specifically it is concerned with the timing of the data at the center of k-space.

BolusTrak

Name for *bolus tracking* on Philips systems.

Bolus tracking

MR angiography technique, which monitors the passage of the contrast agent using rapid 2D imaging in order to initiate the accurate timing of a subsequent sequence. The initiation may be automatic or is more often manually performed. Historically referred to as "MR fluoroscopy" it is also called BolusTrak on Philips systems, CARE bolus (Siemens), Fluorotrigger or SMART prep (GE), FLUTE (Hitachi) and Visual Prep (Toshiba) (Fig. 6).

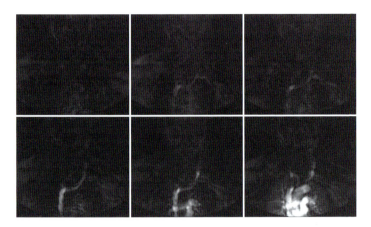

FIGURE 6 A series of images (*left to right, top to bottom*) taken from a *bolus tracking* sequence and used to monitor the arrival of contrast

Bone imaging

The increasing use of MRI to study both the mechanical structure (bone quantity) and the soft-tissue signal of the marrow (bone quality). Spatial resolutions of between 50 and 200 μm are now possible with clinical high field systems and dedicated coils allowing trabecular detail to be investigated. In addition the bone marrow quality can be examined in terms of fat content (see *fat fraction*) (Fig. 7).

Bonferroni correction

Statistical adjustment of some probability statement to account for multiple comparisons of data. For example if 20 tests are carried out with $p = 0.05$ significance level then on average one test will demonstrate an erroneous significance by chance ($1/20 = 0.05$). The correction accounts for this by dividing the single test *p-value* by the number of tests. In fMRI this is equivalent to dividing the p value, by the number of pixels.

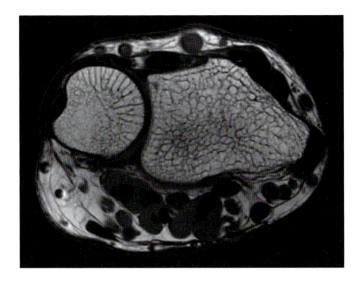

FIGURE 7 *Bone imaging.* Wrist image acquired at 3.0 T with 180 μm in-plane resolution

See also *statistical errors*

References

Everitt BS. Medical statistics from A to Z. Cambridge: Cambridge University Press; 2003. ISBN: 0521532043

Bore

Referring to the overall dimension of the enclosed space within the MR scanner. More specifically this is termed the patient bore, to distinguish the bore width of the final system from the diameter of the main windings which are around 1 m. Traditionally, higher fields have meant an increased length and reduced diameter bore. However modern technology has meant that 3.0 T systems now have similar dimensions to 1.5 T systems of only a few years ago and what constitutes long bore and *short bore* is less well defined. Typical whole-body scanners have a patient bore of around 50–60 cm diameter (see *wide bore*) and are typically around 1.25–1.9 m in length.

See also *short bore*

Bore liner

The use of a plastic insert between patient and scanner bore to reduce *acoustic noise*. Accounts for a noise reduction of between 10 and 15 dB.

Bounce-point artifact

The phenomenon observed in *inversion recovery* where two tissues with different T_1 values recover to the same magnitude either side of the transverse plane so that they appear *isointense* in the final image. They can only be distinguished at a common boundary due to the signal void caused by cancelation of equally negative and positive signal.

Bound protons

The opposite to mobile or *free protons* (e.g., water, CSF). Large macromolecules such as proteins form a hydration layer of tightly bound water molecules. This reduces *molecular tumbling rates* and increases *correlation times*. T_1 values are long but corresponding T_2 values are extremely short so that they are "invisible" on MR images. These molecules may be investigated using *magnetization transfer* imaging.

Box car

A type of fMRI *paradigm* involving regular on and off stimulus periods, typically lasting 20–30 s each. More sophisticated studies use *event related* schemes involving more than one stimulus presentation. The stimulus waveform can be correlated with the pixel values to produce an *activation map*. Often this square shaped waveform is first convolved with an appropriate *hemodynamic response function* to make it more realistic.

BPH

Abbreviation for Benign Prostatic Hyperplasia. Common benign disease usually found in the central gland of the prostate. It is characterized by mixed signal changes on T_2-weighted images (shown in Fig. 26) and can cause either an increase or decrease in the levels of *citrate* seen on MRS. This makes it difficult to distinguish from prostate cancer.

BPP equation

See *Bloembergen, Purcell and Pound equation.*

BRACE

Acronym for BReast Acquisition CorrEction. Siemens post-processing application which provides 3D motion correction to compensate for patient movement in dynamic contrast enhanced imaging of the breast.

See also *registration*.

Brachytherapy

A form of *radiotherapy* where a sealed radioactive source is either permanently or temporarily placed inside the patient using applicators. The method is increasingly utilizing MRI in the planning stage to deliver more conformal doses. This requires the use of *MR compatible* applicators which will create a *susceptibility artifact*.

See also Fig. 56.

BRAVO

Acronym for BRAin VOlume imaging. A fast 3D volume gradient-echo sequence from GE with inversion preparation and using *parallel imaging* to acquire images with excellent spatial resolution in reasonably short scan times.

See also *inversion recovery*.

BREASE

Acronym from BREAst Spectroscopy Examination. A single voxel spectroscopy technique from GE based on the *PRESS* localisation sequence and also using *TE averaging*.

Breast coil

RF coil specifically designed to image the breast. The simplest design consists of two plastic formed wells containing two surface coils. More complicated open designs exist with at least four coils and an opening in between allowing access for minor interventional procedures.

See also *interventional device*.

Breast imaging

See *MR Mammography*.

Breath hold

The method of utilizing very short scan times so that it is possible for the patient to hold their breath. The patients are asked to breathe normally and then hold on exhalation, reducing *motion artifacts* caused by respiration. The verbal instructions to the patient are now usually automated on modern systems. An example image that has been acquired in a single breath hold is shown in Fig. 35.

Bright blood

Images where the blood signal is *hyperintense*. See *white blood*.

Bright fat

The characteristic high signal appearance of fat on T_2-weighted *FSE* images due to breakdown of *J-coupling* effects in the *lipid* molecule caused by the rapid succession of RF pulses.

See also *DIET*.

Broca's area

Part of the frontal lobe of the brain responsible for the production of speech (the motor speech area).

See also *Wernicke's area*.

Brodmann areas

Designation of specific parts of the brain based on their function. In his original work in 1909 Brodmann distinguished each part by the visual appearance under a microscope. Often used in reporting *fMRI* activation regions.

See also *Talairach space*.

Bruker

Swiss-based MRI vendor now operating as Bruker BioSpin. Their systems are principally high field and small bore size magnets for use in research laboratories for small animal and pre-clinical MRI and MRS, although customized whole-body magnets are also available. Magnets range from 4.7 up to 11.7 T (see Fig. 61) with corresponding imaging sizes of 20–7 cm.

www.bruker-biospin.com

BSP

Annotation on a *DICOM* image meaning Blood SuPpression has been used.

"Burnt-in" pixels

Expression relating to the alteration of pixel intensity values to reflect some underlying property. Commonly used as a method of "hard-coding" an *overlay* into an image so it can be used in standard *DICOM* format.

Burst imaging

A type of ultra-fast imaging sequence with *single-shot* capabilities similar to *EPI*. It is characterized by a series of regularly spaced RF pulses of very low flip angle. These are acquired in the presence of the frequency encoding gradient followed by a 180° RF pulse which refocuses these into a train of echoes in the presence of a second gradient. Compared to EPI, single shot mode takes about twice as long. The application of a constant gradient rather than rapidly switching gradients as in EPI, makes it less noisy and it has been used in auditory fMRI and studies of sleep. The original sequence used around 64 pulses with <1° flip angle producing inherently low *SNR*. More recent implementations have attempted to improve SNR for clinical use.

References

Doran SJ, et al. Burst imaging-can it ever be useful in the clinic? Concepts Magn Reson Part A Bridg. 2005; 26:11–34

Buscopan

A commercial drug often administered to reduce *peristaltic motion.*

Byte

A unit of binary data storage. One byte is equal to 8 bits which are assigned values of 1,2,4…128 giving a range of numbers that can be stored from 0 to 255. Four bytes is usually referred to as a word. Commonly image data is stored as a 16 bit short integer representation (or 2 bytes). This gives a possible signal intensity range from 0 to 65,535. On PC and Unix workstations the magnitude of the left or right byte is different. This is referred to as either little or big endian.

Common data types you may come across are integers and floats. Integers (whole numbers) are typically stored in 2 or 4 bytes, (the former classified as a short integer). These can be unsigned (as in image data) or signed, in which case the last bit is reserved for the sign so that a two-byte number is then restricted to a range of –32,768 to +32,768. Decimal numbers are called floats and represent the number and its exponent in 4 bytes. Double precision floats are allocated 8 bytes (two words). A kilobyte (KB) is defined as 2^{10} bytes or 1,024 bytes and should not be confused with kilobit (kb).

See also *bit.*

C

Cable loss

The loss of signal in an RF coil, which results from an impedance mismatch between the coil and the connecting cable. A
correction factor is used in each coil configuration file of the
scanner to account for this loss.

Cadstream

Post-processing software for the analysis of (breast) *dynamic
contrast enhancement* data.

CAL

Annotation on a *DICOM* image indicating a reference or
CALibration image.

Carbogen

A mixture of air composed of 95% O_2 and 5% CO_2. It is used
to study perfusion via *BOLD* effects and also in *ventilation
imaging*.

Carbon

The commonly occurring isotope of carbon (^{12}C) is not MR
visible. However, ^{13}C is MR visible with a chemical shift range
of 200 ppm and a resonant frequency at 1.5 T of 16.1 MHz. Its
weak MR signal can be increased by a factor of 10,000 by the
process of *hyperpolarisation*.

MR properties of ^{13}C:
Spin quantum number = 1/2
Sensitivity = 0.0159
Natural abundance = 1.11%
Gyromagnetic ratio = 10.70 MHz T^{-1}.

Cardiac MRI

The increased use of MRI to provide both anatomical and functional images of the heart. Modern MR scanners with faster gradients, improved *cardiac gating* and dedicated RF coils have meant that cardiac MRI is now performed routinely. Techniques include *cine* MRI, *spin tagging* and myocardial *perfusion imaging*. Traditionally the latter has only been possible with nuclear medicine (e.g., PET). Instead, dynamic contrast enhanced MRI can be used to reveal ischemic regions as signal defects. Imaging following the administration of a suitable *stress-perfusion agent* permits the examination of infarcts more readily (Fig. 8).

See also *delayed contrast enhancement* and *MR Echo*.

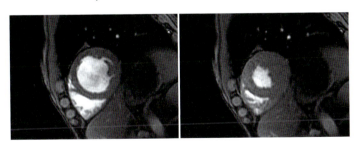

FIGURE 8 *Cardiac MRI*. Short axis views of the left ventricle during diastole (*left*) and systole (*right*). Liney G. MRI in clinical practice. London: Springer; 2006, p. 104.

Cardiac gating

See *ECG gating*.

CARE bolus

Siemens version of *bolus tracking* used in MR angiography which utilizes *key-hole imaging*. The acronym stands for Combine Applications to Reduce Exposure.

Carr-Purcell

Historic name (usually abbreviated to CP) for the basic multiple spin-echo sequence used for measuring T_2. Errors in the flip angle of the nominal $180°$ *refocusing pulse* accumulate with successive echoes leading to an underestimation of T_2. This was subsequently corrected in the modified *CPMG* sequence.

References

Carr HY, Purcell EM. Effects of diffusion on free precession in nuclear magnetic resonance experiments. Phys Rev. 1954;94:630–638

Cartesian

Referring to a rectangular co-ordinate system where a point is defined by its position from two perpendicular axes. Named after the mathematician Descartes. The term is often used in MRI to distinguish normal *k-space trajectory* from *radial k-space*.

Cartigram

Name for GE's T_2 mapping sequence utilizing eight echoes in a multi-echo FSE sequence aimed at cartilage imaging.

CASL

Abbreviation for Continuous *Arterial Spin Labeling*.

CC

Annotation on a *DICOM* image meaning Cardiac Compensation (or gating).

CD

Abbreviation for Compact Disc. Data archiving medium, which is PC compatible. Typically holds 650 MB of images or screen-shot data. Modern scanners now have on-board CD writing capability with images being stored in *DICOM* format often with some proprietary reading software.

See also *DAT*.

CENTRA

Abbreviation of Contrast ENhanced Timing Robust Angiography. Philips contrast-enhanced MRA sequence. Unlike conventional *centric k-space* acquisitions, samples are randomly acquired from a central disk portion during the arterial phase and then proceed to the outer k-space.

References

Willinek WA, et al. Randomly segmented central k-space ordering in high-spatial resolution contrast-enhanced MR angiography of the supraaortic arteries: initial experience. Radiology. 2002;225:583–588

Central k-space

The inner portion of *k-space* data corresponding to the bulk of image signal. Also referred to as *low order phase*.

Central point artifact

An image artifact resulting in a bright spot at the center of an image. It is caused by a DC offset in the receiver. Occasionally very stable RF interference may appear as a spot on the image rather than the more usual line (see *zipper artifact*).

Center frequency

The resonant frequency that the RF coil is tuned to during the pre-scan routine. The center frequency is nominally set to the water peak. From this other frequencies and bandwidths can be properly assigned, for example the fat peak in *CHESS*. The center frequency should be stable over time (see *field stability*).

See also *Larmor frequency*.

Centric k-space filling

Conventionally k-space is filled in a *sequential* or linear fashion (i.e., highest negative gradient steps through to highest positive steps). In centric filling (or ordering), the center of k-space, corresponding to the low positive and negative phase steps, is filled first. This is also referred to as low-high filling. The opposite of this is reverse or concentric filling. The filling order becomes important in certain situations, for example in *gating* or *contrast-enhanced MRA*.

See also *k-space ordering* and *k-space trajectory*.

Cerebral blood flow (volume)

Two *perfusion* parameters specifically related to imaging in the brain. Cerebral blood flow (CBF) is defined as the perfusion rate per unit mass of tissue. It is related to the peak signal loss in a dynamic susceptibility contrast scan (see *perfusion imaging*). Cerebral blood volume (CBV) is the total blood volume in the region of interest and is estimated by the *area under the curve* (or negative enhancement integral). CBV is affected by many pathological conditions.

CBV is related to CBF by:

$$CBV = CBF \times MTT.$$

where MTT is the mean *transit time*.

To gain an accurate measure of CBF the *arterial input function* (AIF) needs to be deconvolved from the tissue signal.

References

Calamante F, Thomas DL, Pell GS, et al. Measuring cerebral blood flow using magnetic resonance imaging techniques. J Cereb Blood Flow Metab. 1999;19:701–735

Cerebrospinal fluid

Usually abbreviated to CSF. This is fluid that circulates around the spinal cord and brain and acts as both protection and nourishment. Its long T_1 and T_2 relaxation times give it a characteristic appearance (see Figs. 92 and 94). The high signal on T_2-weighted images may be suppressed using techniques such as *FLAIR*.

CHARM

Acronym for CHunk Acquisition and Reconstruction Method. A Philips contrast-enhanced MRA sequence, which acquires overlapping volumes and then uses a weighting algorithm to reduce the *venetian blind artifact*.

Chemical shift

The shift or change in resonant frequency of a particular nuclear spin due to different chemical environments. It forms the basis of MR spectroscopy through the identification of molecules depending on their chemical shift. Specifically a molecular electron cloud shields the nucleus from the full extent of B_0 reducing the field as:

$$B' = B_0(1 - \sigma)$$

where σ is the *shielding constant*. The effect was first observed in metals by Knight giving it an historic name of Knight shift.

See also *PPM*.

Chemical shift artifact

An artifact with the characteristic appearance of bright and dark bands on opposite sides of an object or tissue and propagating in the frequency encoding direction. It is due to the mismapping of fat and water, which coexist in the object (or patient) but become spatially distinct in the image. The basis for the effect is the finite frequency range used to assign to each pixel and the chemical shift between fat and water. The artifact may be reduced by increasing the receiver *bandwidth*, in order to accommodate this frequency difference, which is equal to 220 Hz at 1.5 T. The artifact is worse at high field as the frequency difference increases.

The chemical shift is so large in *EPI* that fat suppression or water-only selective RF pulses must be employed. Unusually in EPI, the artifact is present in the phase encoding direction.

In spectroscopy, the chemical shift causes a misregistration of the fat and water voxel position which may be significant for small voxels. This is sometimes incorrectly referred to as *voxel bleeding* (Fig. 9).

See also *variable BW* and *chemical shift ("of the second kind")*.

Chemical shift imaging

Also more usually abbreviated to CSI. Term that can be used to describe techniques that produce separate fat and water-only images e.g., *DIXON, IDEAL*.

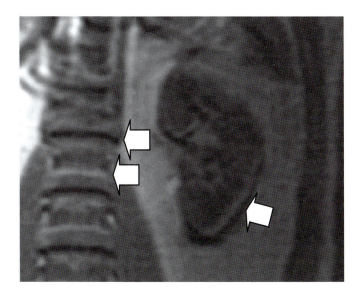

FIGURE 9 Dark and bright signal can be seen on opposite sides of the vertebra and kidney characteristic of *chemical shift artifact*. Frequency direction is top to bottom. Liney G. MRI in clinical practice. London: Springer; 2006, p. 47

It is also used to describe multi-voxel spectroscopy techniques, the spectra from which may be turned into a low resolution image based on *chemical shift*, although this is increasingly referred to as MR Spectroscopic Imaging or *MRSI*.

Chemical shift ("of the second kind")

An artifact which produces signal voids arising from phase differences between fat and water. Unlike frequency-related chemical shift, it appears in both directions and this symmetrical appearance gives it an alternative name of relief artifact. It can be eliminated by acquiring the image at specific echo times so that the fat and water signals are in phase (approximately 4.2 ms at 1.5 T). Most scanners permit the user to select the echo time to be either "in-phase" or "out-of-phase" (Fig. 10).

See also *fat-water in-phase*.

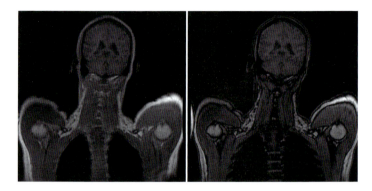

FIGURE 10 *Chemical shift ('of the second kind')*. Images acquired with (*left*) in-phase and (*right*) out-of-phase echo times. The out-of-phase image displays signal voids due to the fat-water signal cancelation

CHESS

Acronym for CHEmical Shift Saturation. A method of *fat suppression* where a narrow bandwidth RF pulse (typically 50 Hz) is centerd on the fat resonance and is used to excite the fat signal only. This is then dephased by gradients prior to the acquisition of the imaging sequence leaving only the water signal remaining. The technique is also referred to as Fat Sat (or Fat Saturation) (Fig. 11).

Chess (or checker) board

A commonly used visual *paradigm* in functional MRI. A chess board pattern is displayed to the patient and the black and white squares alternate at a certain frequency to stimulate the visual cortex.

Chiller

Large refrigeration unit outside the MRI building used to provide a cold water supply for the *cold head*.

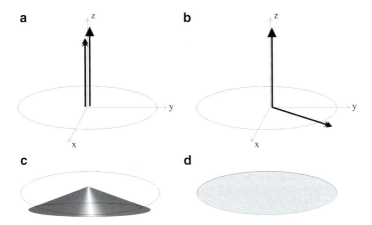

FIGURE 11 *CHESS* fat suppression. (**a**) Fat (*double arrow head*) and water initially in alignment with B_0. (**b**) The fat is flipped slightly into the –z direction where it is dephased by gradients (**c**). In the subsequent imaging sequence only water is left (**d**). Liney G. MRI in clinical practice. London: Springer; 2006, p. 9

Choline

Choline containing compounds demonstrate a peak in proton spectroscopy at 3.22 ppm. The signal comes from glycero-phosphocholine, phosphocholine (also observed in phosphorus MRS) and a small amount of free choline (see Fig. 53). It is indicative of cell turnover, and its elevation is thought to be a marker of cancer. Particular attention is paid to the choline peak in breast cancer spectroscopy as it is not normally detectable in healthy tissue (Fig. 12).

See also *MR mammography* and *GRACE*.

$$HO-CH_2-CH_2-\overset{CH_3}{\underset{CH_3}{\overset{|}{\underset{\|}{N}}}}-CH_3$$

FIGURE 12 The chemical structure of *choline*

Chunk

An alternative name for an imaging *slab*.

CIA

Abbreviation for Contrast free Improved Angiography. A non-contrast enhanced MRA sequence from Toshiba. Other similar sequences include InHance (GE), TRANCE (Philips), NATIVE (Siemens), and VASC (Hitachi).

Cine

1. Referring to the displaying and viewing of sequential images in a movie loop. Images may be viewed in temporal or spatial order and can be played back in a loop or yo-yo back and forth. Useful for displaying *dynamic contrast enhancement* images or studying physiological motion e.g., in cardiac MRI.
2. A term used generally to refer to any fast multiphase technique that is used to acquire images of physiological motion. It is almost exclusively used to refer to cardiac imaging. The technique can be used in order to measure the end diastolic and end systolic volumes, from which the relative volume increase (or *ejection fraction*) is calculated.

Circularity

A measurement of shape that is defined as the ratio of the standard deviation to the mean distance of each point on the perimeter to the center of the shape. A perfect circle will produce a value of zero.

See also *morphological descriptors*.

Circularly polarized

Another term for *quadrature* detection and/or transmission RF coils.

CISS

Acronym for Constructive Interference Steady State. A Siemens sequence which produces strongly T_2-weighted images by combining two *FISP* echoes. Often used in *MR Cisternography*, but is now largely redundant since the introduction of 3D FSE sequences.

See also *steady state*.

Citrate

Metabolite that occurs in uniquely high concentrations in the prostate gland. It is an important marker of prostate cancer, with levels being reduced in malignancy. Its proton MRS peak is seen at 2.6 ppm (see Fig. 99). It is designated an *AB system*, with a chemical shift separation of 15.4 Hz and a coupling constant of 7.8 Hz (Fig. 13).

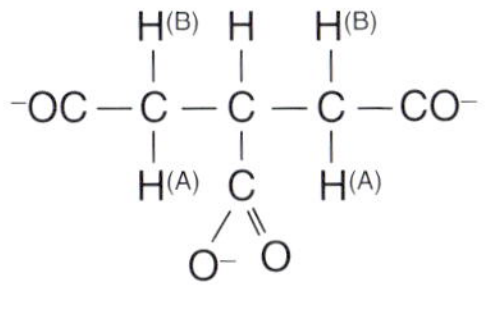

FIGURE 13 The chemical structure of *citrate* with the A and B protons identified

References

Schick F, Bongers H, Kurz S, Jung WI, Pfeffer M, Lutz O. Localised proton MR spectroscopy of citrate in vitro and of the human prostate in vivo at 1.5 T. Magn Reson Med. 1993;29:38–43

Claustrophobia

The fear of enclosed spaces which is sometimes encountered by patients having an MRI scan due to its confined nature. Modern systems are wider and shorter than those used previously and this helps reduce the incidence although the number of patients affected can still be up to 20%. Patient positioning is also an important factor (e.g., supine, prone, head first entry). Methods of reducing its effects include a *head coil* mirror, bore lighting, air-flow, and music (usually *feet first entry* only) or use of an *open scanner*. In extreme cases a small amount of sedative may be required (e.g., benzodiazepine).

CLEAR

Acronym meaning Constant LEvel AppeaRance.
  See also *coil uniformity correction*.

Cliavist

Another brand name for the contrast agent *Resovist*.

Closed scanner

The conventional horizontal tunnel-like *bore* design of most MRI systems (for example Fig. 48).
  See also *open scanner*.

CNR

Abbreviation for *contrast-to-noise ratio*.

Coil

See *RF coil*.

Coil uniformity correction

A method of improving image uniformity by correcting for the inhomogeneous reception profile of RF coils. It usually involves weighting the image by an appropriate sensitivity function, which is often empirically determined from a calibration scan e.g., a *proton density weighted* (low contrast) image. GE offer two methods known as *SCIC* and *PURE*. On Philips systems there are three levels of correction: strong, weak and *CLEAR* (Fig. 14).

See also B_1 *inhomogeneity*.

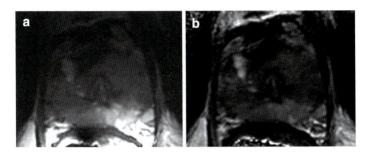

FIGURE 14 (**a**) A prostate image obtained with the endorectal coil and demonstrating signal flare close to the coil with rapid signal drop off further away. In (**b**) the author's own *coil uniformity correction* has been applied and the image uniformity is improved

References

Liney GP, Turnbull LW, Knowles AJ. A simple method for the correction of endorectal surface coil inhomogeneity in prostate imaging. J Magn Reson Imaging. 1998;8:994–997

Cold head

The device that sits on top of the magnet and accepts heat from the vaporizing helium from the *cryostat* in order to recondense it (see Fig. 48). This heat is transferred by fluid to the cold head compressor (a *heat exchanger*) situated outside the scan room where it is cooled by water from a *chiller*.

Colored orientation map

A type of parameter map used in *DTI* indicating the direction of diffusion by color. A separate color is used to represent each orthogonal direction so that 3D information is conveyed on a 2D image. In addition, the brightness of the color is often scaled by the value of the *fractional anisotropy* of each pixel (Fig. 15).

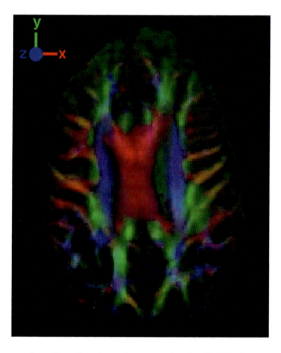

FIGURE 15 A *colored orientation map* in the brain demonstrating fiber tracts running left-to-right (*red*), anterior-to-posterior (*green*) and head-to-foot (*blue*)

Combidex

Alternative commercial name for the contrast agent *Sinerem*.

Commissural fibers

Type of *white matter fibers* that connect parts of the brain from one hemisphere to the other. Important groups are the corpus callosum (literally hard body) and the anterior commisure and posterior commissure which are used in fMRI registration (see *Talairach space*).

Complexity

A measure used to describe the irregularity of a region-of-interest. It is defined as the square of the perimeter divided by the surface area, with a circle being equal to 4π.

See also *morphological descriptors*.

Composite pulses

A series of RF pulses that are concatenated to improve their overall utilization. A common example is a *binomial pulse*.

Conjugate symmetry

The property of *k-space* which means that the data values on one side of k-space are identical to the values at their mirrored location through the origin:

$$S\left(k_{PE},k_{FE}\right)= S^*\left(-k_{PE},-k_{FE}\right)$$

This permits the interpolation of missing data points when only part of k-space data is acquired (see *partial Fourier, partial echo*). It is also referred to as *hermitian* symmetry. The above equation means that a minimum of half of k-space must be collected. In practice slightly more than 50% of k-space is acquired and the extra data can be used to correct for any phase errors.

Constant EPI

An *EPI* sequence where the phase encoding gradient is continually applied producing a zig-zag *k-space trajectory*.
    See also *spiral EPI* and *blipped EPI*.

Contiguous

Referring to adjacent imaging slices with no gaps. This can lead to *cross-excitation* due to overlapping slice profiles if the slices are not *interleaved*.

Continuous wave NMR

A technique whereby resonance is achieved by applying a continuous sweep of radiofrequency.
    See also *adiabatic pulse*.

Contraindications

Referring to the presentation of a patient which prevents the acquisition of the MRI examination. For example patients with a *pacemaker* or certain implants etc.
    See also *projectile* and *pregnancy*.

Contrast

The visual difference in signal intensities between adjacent structures on an image. It may be quantified by expressing the difference in signal from two regions divided by the summation or measuring *contrast-to-noise ratio*.

Contrast agents

A substance, (an exogenous chemical agent), which is used to alter the signal properties within the image. The majority of contrast agents usually shorten relaxation times but spin-density agents also exists (e.g., glucose, deuterium oxide).

Relaxation shortening agents can be subdivided into *paramagnetic* and superparamagnetic iron oxide types (see *SPIO*). These agents work by creating a local field variation in their immediate vicinity causing signal changes.

The paramagnetic types cause a T_1 shortening or a positive enhancement effect. The exact nature of the signal change depends on the *relaxivity* of the agent but also on the concentration. At extremely high concentrations (>10 times the normal dose) T_2 effects dominate (see *pseudolayering*).

The most common paramagnetic agents are the extracellular *gadolinium*-based agents. Others include albumin-binding agents (to create a *blood pool agent*) and non-gadolinium agents e.g., *manganese*.

SPIO agents shorten T_2 and therefore cause a negative enhancement effect.

Agents are typically administered intravenously followed by a *saline flush* although *enteral contrast agents* can also be used.

See also *Gd-DTPA*, *USPIO* and *endogenous contrast.*

Contrast enhanced

Referring to images which are acquired following the administration of a contrast agent to improve signal differences in tissues. The majority of studies utilize T_1-weighted images, which demonstrate increased signal in the presence of a positive contrast agent. It is particularly useful in the study of tumors, which demonstrate a preferential uptake of these agents due to *angiogenesis* (Fig. 16).

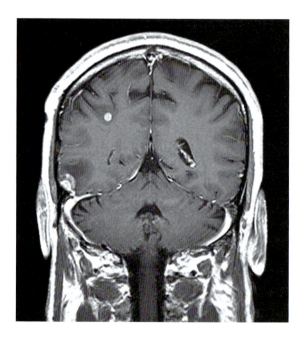

FIGURE 16 This *contrast enhanced* image demonstrates two metastatic tumors. Liney G. MRI in clinical practice. London: Springer; 2006, p. 68

Contrast-enhanced MRA

The use of MR contrast agents to directly image the vascular tree. The main advantage over other techniques (e.g., *TOF*) is that there is no reliance on saturation effects, so that slice thickness and flow orientation is not a limiting factor. At present most agents in use are extracellular in nature which causes an unwanted background enhancement. This is improved with either accurate *bolus timing* or use of specific *blood pool agents* (Fig. 17).

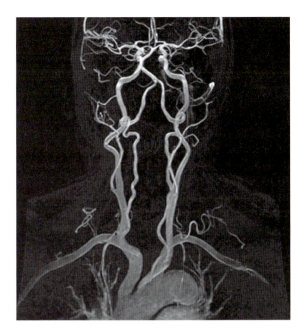

FIGURE 17 A *contrast enhanced-MRA* example demonstrating coverage from the aortic arch to the intra-cranial vessels. Liney G. MRI in clinical practice. London: Springer; 2006, p. 113

References

Prince MR, Yucel EK, Kaufman JA, et al. Dynamic gadolinium-enhanced 3D abdominal MR angiography. J Magn Reson Imaging. 1993;3:877–881

Contrast phantom

A specifically designed test object for examining the contrast properties of different image sequences. Usually consists of multiple compartments with materials of varying relaxation times.

See also *gel phantoms* and *quality assurance*.

Contrast-to-noise ratio

A quantitative measure of the relative signal-to-noise differences from two different regions. It is defined as:

$$CNR = (S_1 - S_2)/\sigma$$

where S_1 and S_2 are the mean signal intensity values from the two regions and σ is the standard deviation of the background signal or noise (see *SNR*). This is sometimes also referred to as the signal difference to noise ratio (SDNR).

A related measurement is contrast factor which is the signal differences divided by the summation of the two signals.

Contrast factor

See *contrast-to-noise ratio*.

Control room

The secure area from where the scanner is operated by radiographic staff and some image processing and archiving may also take place.

See also *scan room*.

Controlled mode

A designated operational level of the scanner where any patient effects should be mild and transient.

See also *bio-effects*, *normal mode*, *research mode* and *safety limits*.

Convexity

A measure used to describe the irregularity of a region-of-interest. It is calculated by enclosing the region with straight lines to form the smallest area possible. The convexity is then the proportion of the original area inside this new area. Highly spiculated areas (e.g., tumors) will have low values of convexity.

See also *morphological descriptors*.

Copper

A ductile and conductive metal which is used in the construction of the scan room to provide *RF shielding*.

Copper is also used in the form of aqueous solutions of copper sulfate to alter the relaxation properties of water in phantoms. The T_1 and T_2 *relaxivity* values for copper are similar (for the Cu^{2+} ion this is approximately 0.7 mM^{-1}s^{-1}).

See also *doping*.

Copper sulfate

See *copper*.

Coronal

Referring to the imaging plane, which divides the subject into anterior and posterior parts i.e., the slice selection is in the y direction and the in-plane directions run right-to-left and head-to-foot. It is also known as the frontal plane (Fig. 18).

See also *sagittal*, *axial* and *oblique*.

Corduroy artifact

Alternative name for *herringbone artifact*.

Correlation coefficient

A statistical measure which indicates how closely related two sets of data are. It is particularly useful in *fMRI* analysis in

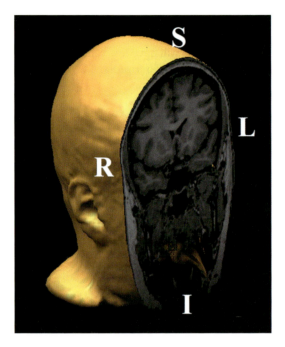

FIGURE 18 A 3D reconstruction of a brain volume which has been sliced in the *coronal* plane. The image is labeled to indicate the Superior, Inferior, Left and Right directions

order to compare pixel intensity changes with the stimulus pattern. Values range from −1 to 1, with the extreme values indicating a perfect correlation (the sign indicating the direction of the relationship), and zero indicates no correlation. Results are usually reported together with a *P-value*.

See also *activation map*.

Correlation time

The average time interval before a molecule collides (denoted τ_c). Solids have long correlation times whereas values in liquids and gases are shorter. Higher temperatures reduce this value. It is related to *molecular tumbling rate*.

See also *Bloembergen, Pound and Purcell equation*.

COSMIC

Pulse sequence acronym for Coherent Oscillatory State acquisition for the Manipulation of Imaging Contrast. A GE sequence that is *FIESTA* based but has modified *elliptic centric k-space filling* and oscillates the flip angle to move in and out of *steady state* quickly allowing T_1 recovery. It provides high signal-to-noise in bone, muscle and cartilage and is particularly useful in cervical nerve roots and intervertebral discs.

COSY

Acronym for COrrelation SpectroscopY. A common implementation of proton 2D spectroscopy. Two 90° pulses are used (referred to as preparation and mixing pulses) with the time interval varied in a series of experiments. This produces spectroscopy data that can be displayed as contour plots on two axes. Conventional 1D spectra are usually shown on each axis to provide a reference. The plot reveals diagonal peaks and cross peaks with the latter indicating which protons exhibit *J-coupling* (Fig. 19).

See also *Heteronuclear correlation spectroscopy* and *NOESY.*

References

Keeler J. Understanding NMR spectroscopy. Chichester: Wiley; 2005. ISBN. 0470017872

Cortical flattening

A post-processing method used in functional MRI (see *fMRI*), which removes the undulations of the cerebral cortex to accurately localize the region of activation.

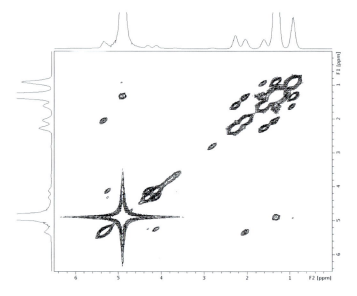

FIGURE 19 A *COSY* plot in a phantom containing cream and demonstrating both diagonal and cross-peaks

Cortical inflation

A functional MRI (see *fMRI*) post-processing method, which involves transposing image data onto a standardized brain volume for cross-study comparisons.

CPMG

Abbreviation for the Carr-Purcell-Meiboom-Gill sequence used to measure T_2. The basic unit (Carr-Purcell or CP) is a multiple spin-echo sequence in which signal decay is measured at different echo times (*TE*). In the modified sequence (CPMG), the phase (direction) of the 180° refocusing pulse is alternated to prevent compounding errors in the flip angle so that every even echo is accurate.

References

Meiboom S, Gill D. Modified sin-echo method for measuring nuclear relaxation times. Rev Sci Instrum. 1958;29:688–691

Craniocaudal

Another name for the head-to-foot or superior-inferior direction.

Creatine

A proton metabolite that together with phosphocreatine is observed at 3.02 and 3.94 ppm. The creatine peak has been used as a constant signal reference but it has also been shown to decrease in tumors (see Fig. 53) (Fig. 20).

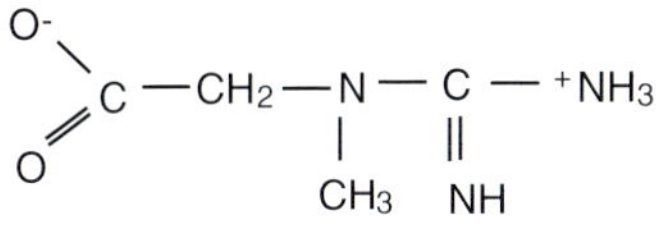

FIGURE 20 The chemical structure of *creatine*

Critical temperature

The temperature below which certain materials become superconducting. This is typically approaching absolute zero, (e.g., 4 K or −269°C for *niobium-titanium*).

See also *superconducting magnet*.

Cross-excitation

Refers to the erroneous excitation of an adjacent slice due to an imperfect *slice profile*. The problem can be reduced by using an *interleaved* slice acquisition or including a sufficient *slice gap* in-between slices (usually 10% of the nominal slice thickness is required). Often confused with *cross talk*, although this is strictly speaking a different effect.

Cross peak

See *COSY*.

Cross talk

The exchange of energy between spins in adjacent slices due to T_1 relaxation.

Crusher gradients

The specific application of gradients in order to eliminate unwanted signal by deliberately causing it to dephase. These are also sometimes known as killer gradients.

See also *spoiling*.

Cryogens

The liquids (usually helium) used within the scanner *cryostat*, which maintain the *critical temperature* of the superconducting magnet. Earlier scanners also used liquid nitrogen. The cryostat is vented at the top of the scanner to ensure the safe removal of the cryogens in the advent of a *quench*. The degree to which the cryogens need to be replenished is given by the *boil-off* rate.

Cryogen free

Novel magnets that utilize high temperature superconducting materials which can be cooled directly by the *cold head* and do not require *cryogens*.

Cryoshielding

The method of reducing the *boil-off* rate of the *cryogens* by externally cooling the *cryostat*.

Cryostat

The unit used to hold the superconducting magnet in a cryogen bath ensuring minimal evaporation or *boil-off*. It has an outer vacuum compartment which is separated from the inner cryogen container by a shield which is externally cooled by a cryocooler or *cold head*. Older systems used liquid nitrogen as this shield around the helium container.

See also *cryogens* and *cryoshielding*.

Cryotherapy

Treatment of tumors by freezing, which can be performed under MR guidance.

See also *MR thermometry*.

C-SCAN

A dedicated extremity scanner utilizing a 0.2 T *permanent magnet*. It requires no RF shielding and can be sited in a small area such as an office workspace using a normal power supply. Other larger systems include the E-scan and G-scan, which can rotate 90° to perform *positional MRI*.

http://www.grucox.com/

CSF

Abbreviation for *Cerebrospinal fluid*.

CSI

Abbreviation for *Chemical Shift Imaging*.

CSPAMM

Abbreviation for Complementary *SPAMM*. An additional modification to the SPAMM sequence which involves the subtraction of positive and negative grid lines in order to improve the contrast of the cardiac tagging.

CT

Abbreviation for Computer Tomography (also formally known as CAT or Computer Assisted Tomography). A widespread medical imaging method utilizing X-rays to obtain multi-planar images, first used in 1973. Unlike MRI, it has little soft-tissue contrast. It is still the modality of choice in certain areas, for example in *radiotherapy planning* where the signal attenuation is used to estimate electron density, or in trauma or spinal-injuries where analysis of bone is crucial.

CTL coil

A type of RF *surface coil* array with selectable elements for imaging either the Cervical, Thoracic or Lumbar spine.

CUBE

A GE sequence (and not an acronym). A 3D fast spin-echo sequence which uses an optimized train of refocusing RF pulses allowing an extended echo train. It provides *isotropic* resolution, reduces blurring and lowers *SAR*. Equivalent sequences include *SPACE* (Siemens) and *VISTA* (Philips).

D

DAC

Abbreviation for Digital-to-Analog Converter. This is hardware which turns the digital signal generated by the *double balanced mixer* into an analog signal for RF transmission.

See also *ADC*.

Daily QA

A basic routine quality assurance protocol usually involving a visual check of a manufacturer's phantom prior to clinical imaging.

See also *quality assurance*.

DANTE

Acronym for Delays Alternating with Nutation for Tailored Excitation. This refers to a type of sequence that utilizes a series of low angle RF excitation pulses. It has been used as a method of *spin-tagging* in cardiac MRI.

See also *DUFIS*.

DAT

A digital tape archiving medium holding approximately 1.3 GB of images. It has largely been phased out in favor of optical discs (*OD*) or CDs.

Data clipping

See *over-ranging*.

Daum needles

Specially coated *MR compatible* biopsy needles used to reduce the *susceptibility artifact*.

db/dt

Pronounced "db by dt." This refers to the rate of change of magnetic field generated by the imaging *gradient* and defined by the *slew rate*. A high value of this improves imaging speed but can lead to *peripheral nerve stimulation*.

DCE

Abbreviation for *Dynamic Contrast Enhancement*.

DCIS

Abbreviation for Ductal Carcinoma In Situ. A type of breast cancer that is particularly difficult to detect and is being increasingly examined with MRI.

DDA

Abbreviation of DiasableD (or DiscardeD) Acquisitions. A GE term for *dummy* acquisitions.

Dead time

The period after the echo time (*TE*) and prior to the application of the next RF excitation pulse. During this time other adjacent slices are excited thereby improving the efficiency of 2D imaging. For example in a spin-echo sequence with TE/

TR = 200 ms/1 s, five (=1,000/200) slices can theoretically be acquired per TR.

Decay

Describing the general loss of MR signal due to *dephasing* effects in the transverse plane.

Decimation

The process of reducing the spatial resolution of an image. It is the opposite of *interpolation*.

DEFAISE

Acronym for the Dual-Echo FAst Interleaved Spin Echo pulse sequence. A variation of the *FAISE* sequence producing two images per repetition time.

Deflection angle test

An ex-vivo method of testing the MR compatibility of non-ferromagnetic or weakly ferromagnetic implants and devices. The object is suspended freely and brought into the scan room to observe the angle it is deflected. Angles less than $45°$ indicate that the force it experiences is no greater than gravity and it is deemed safe.

DEFT

Acronym for the Driven Equilibrium Fourier Transformation sequence.
See also *driven equilibrium.*

Delayed contrast enhancement

A technique used to assess cardiac viability. Dysfunctioning myo-cardium shows up as late hyperenhancement due to its impaired wash-out compared to normal tissue (see *cardiac MRI*).

Another delayed contrast technique is used in cartilage imaging which involves assessing the penetration of gadolinium several hours after its administration. This is used to assess glycosaminoglycan content.

Delay time

See T_{del}.

Delta

Greek letter used in uppercase (Δ) to denote a change in some value and in lowercase (δ) to denote *chemical shift*.

Demodulation

The removal of the RF component of the measured MR signal to leave an audiofrequency (AF) signal. This works by comparing the signal with a sinusoidal pulse at the resonant frequency. The result is then passed onto the analog-to-digital converter (*ADC*) for further processing.

Dephasing

Loss of *phase* coherence of spins due to interaction with neighboring spins (T_2) or inhomogeneities in the magnetic field. The combined effect is described by the relaxation term T_2^*.

Dephasing lobe

Part of the *slice selection* and *frequency encoding* gradient, which is applied with opposite polarity to ensure that there is no net phase change when the remaining part of the gradient is applied. The amplitude (area on a *pulse sequence diagram*) of the lobe is set to half that of the main gradient. Depashing lobes can be on the slice selection gradients in Figs. 27, 36, 44 and 88 and additionally on the frequency encoding gradients in Figs. 44 and 88.

DESS

Acronym for the Double Echo Steady State sequence. This combines a *FISP* echo and a subsequent *PSIF* echo to produce high resolution images with strong fluid signal (i.e., a large T_2-weighting). It is used mainly in orthopedic imaging.

Deuterium

An isotope of *hydrogen* (^2H) containing a proton and neutron and therefore having a mass number of 2. It is MR visible but has an extremely low abundance and sensitivity compared to ^1H.

MR properties of ^2H:

Spin quantum number $= 1$
Sensitivity $= 0.0097$
Natural abundance $= 0.015\%$
Gyromagnetic ratio $= 6.53$ MHz T $^{-1}$

Dewar

The MR-compatible container that is taken into the scan room and used to transport and re-fill the *cryogens*. It contains a vacuum to insulate the contents from the outside (Dewar is named after the inventor of the vacuum flask).

DEXA

Acronym for Dual Energy X-ray Absorptiometry. A method for assessing bone mineral density in the examination of osteoporosis. It has the disadvantage of being a 2D projection technique which cannot separate cortical and trabecular bone. High-resolution MRI is being increasingly used in *bone imaging*, with spatial resolution of between 50 and 200 μm.

Dextran

A polysaccharide used to coat iron-oxide particles in order to create *USPIO* type contrast agents. It is identified as the "tran" part of generic compound names such as Ferucarbotran (*Resovist*) and Ferumoxtran (*Sinerem*).

Diamagnetic

The property of material with a negative *susceptibility* i.e., the magnetic field induced within the material when placed in an external magnetic field (mediated by electrons) acts in the opposite direction. It is present due to unpaired electrons and common examples include water.

See also *paramagnetic* and *magnetization*.

DICOM

Acronym for Digital Imaging and COmmunications in Medicine. An industry standard of medical image format, permitting the ease of data transfer between different proprietary devices. The DICOM standard is an enhancement of the previous ACR-NEMA standards (American College of

Radiology & National Electrical Manufacturers Association).
A DICOM image consists of an image *header* containing tags
or entries of information, which may be interpreted in a
known fashion and is followed by the pixel intensity values.

See http://medical.nema.org

Dielectric constant

See *permittivity*.

Dielectric effect

A resonance effect that is especially seen at high field in
materials with a high dielectric constant or *permittivity*, ε,
(e.g., water with $\varepsilon = 80$). The effect produces a *standing wave
artifact*. It can be reduced in *phantom* imaging by using
smaller diameter test objects or materials with lower permittivity (e.g., *silicon* oil, $\varepsilon = 1–3$) (Fig. 21).

See also B_1 *doming* and *wavelength*.

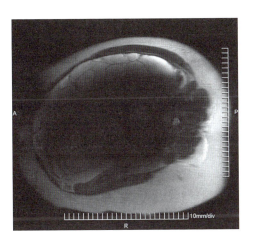

FIGURE 21 An example of gross signal attenuation caused by the
dielectric effect in this image acquired at 3.0 T

References

Tofts PS, Barker GJ, Dean TL, Gallagher H, Gregory AP, Clarke RN. A low dielectric constant customized phantom design to measure RF coil nonuniformity. Magn Reson Imaging. 1997;15:69–75

Dielectric pad

An object containing material with a high dielectric constant, which is appropriately positioned on the patient to improve signal uniformity at high field. It works by taking advantage of the *dielectric effect* in the pad rather than the patient. Often simply a water-filled bag is used, appropriately doped to give it a short T_2 so it does not appear in the image (Fig. 22).

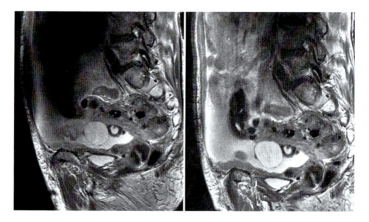

FIGURE 22 This pelvic image acquired at 3.0 T (*left*) demonstrates signal non-uniformity that is rectified when a *dielectric pad* is placed on the abdomen (*right*). Liney G. MRI in clinical practice. London: Springer; 2006, p. 98

DIET

Acronym for the Delayed Interval Echo Train sequence. The use of an increased echo spacing between the first pair of RF pulses in an *FSE* sequence in order to conserve the *J-coupling* effects in fat and therefore create a more spin-echo-like contrast.

See also *bright fat*.

Diffusion

The random movement of molecules also known as Brownian motion. It is characterized by the Einstein equation:

$$<r^2> = 2Dt$$

where $<r^2>$ is the mean-squared displacement, D is the diffusion coefficient and t is the time.

See also *DWI*.

Diffusion ellipsoid

A graphical representation of the diffusion tensor (see *DTI*) which involves drawing ellipsoids at each pixel location in an image. The shape indicates the degree of anisotropy; the size gives the magnitude of diffusion and the orientation demonstrates the preferred diffusion direction. Typically shapes may be spherical (indicating isotropic diffusion in all planes), disc-shaped (isotropic in two planes) or cigar-shaped (a preferred diffusion in one direction).

See also *colored orientation map*.

Diffusion tensor

See *DTI*.

Diffusion tensor spectroscopy

Referring to the particular application of the diffusion tensor for non-water molecules, for example metabolites of the brain such as NAA etc.

Diffusion time

The time between the bipolar gradient pulses used in a typical DWI sequence. By increasing this time it is possible to examine *restricted diffusion*. It is equal to the Δ-δ/3 term in the *b-factor* equation.

Diffusion-weighted imaging

See *DWI*.

Dimeglumine gadopentatate

Chemical name for *Gd-DTPA*. Marketed by Schering as Magnevist.

Dipole

The concept of a north-south magnetic field or *moment* produced by a spinning nucleus.

Dipole–dipole interactions

The interactions between two nuclear spins. The directional nature of a *dipole* means that, depending on the position of one dipole with respect to another, the magnetic field is either augmented or reduced. In a moving water molecule the field can change ±7.0 G. These interactions are the most dominant in causing T_1 and T_2 relaxation.

The magnitude of this effect is given by:

$$3\cos^2\theta - 1$$

where θ is the angle between each dipole. This leads to the so-called *magic-angle effect* at $\theta = 54.7°$ (producing zero interaction).

Another spin interaction, *J-coupling*, refers to interactions between spins of the same molecule via electron cloud distortions.

Dirac's constant

See *h*.

Direction map

See *colored orientation map*.

Discarded data

See *DDA*.

Dispersion

Referring to the separation of adjacent MR Spectroscopy peaks. Dispersion increases linearly with field strength, enabling closely spaced peaks such as glutamate and glutamine (see *Glx*) to become resolved at fields of 3.0 T and above.

See also *chemical shift*.

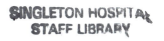

Distance factor

An alternative name given for *slice gap* on Siemens scanners where the separation between slices is given as a percentage of the slice thickness used.

Distortion

Referring to any geometrical differences between the final image and the actual true shape. Distortion is often further classified into *geometric distortion* and *linearity*.

Distortion correction

Application of some method to rectify geometric distortion and non-linearity of a system. Vendors usually provide a 2D correction which is applied automatically (e.g., Gradwarp on GE). Full 3D correction can be made using independent phantom-based mapping which can be used prospectively to restore images.

References

Wang D, Strugnell W, Cowin G, Doddrell DM, Slaughter R. Geometric distortion in clinical MRI systems: part II: correction using a 3D phantom. Magn Reson Imaging. 2004;22:1223–1232

Dixon

A method of *fat suppression* making use of the phase differences between fat and water. Two images are acquired: the first with a suitable echo-time so that fat and water signals are in phase, the second with fat-water out of phase, and a subtraction is subsequently taken. In the three-point Dixon method (see *IDEAL*), a third in-phase image is acquired to correct for B_0 inhomogeneities. On Siemens systems, images are labeled as DIXW and DIXF for water and fat only images respectively.

See also *chemical shift ("of the second kind")* and *OOPS*.

DIXW (DIXF)

See *Dixon*.

DNP

Abbreviation for *Dynamic Nuclear Polarization*.

Dobutamine

A *stress-perfusion agent*.

Doping

The use of a chemical agent to enhance the relaxation rate of water and therefore mimic in vivo signal characteristics in a test object or *phantom*. Common agents include *gadolinium*, *copper*, *nickel*, and *manganese* salts. The main drawback is that their T_1 and T_2 values are similar unlike tissue which has $T_1 > 4 \times T_2$. The exception to this is manganese chloride which has a much longer T_1 compared to T_2. Most compounds will exhibit temperature dependence, particularly copper sulfate.

Some suggested concentrations for aqueous phantom solutions are as follows:

Copper sulfate = 3.15 mM
Nickel chloride = 7.0–10.0 mM
Manganese chloride = 0.14–0.30 mM

Sometimes hydrochloric acid is added to maintain an acidic pH which stops precipitation of the salts. *Sodium chloride* may

also be added to change the conductivity. Finally, preserva-
tives (e.g., sodium azide) may also be included.

See also *relaxivity*.

Dotarem

Commercial name of one of the commonly used gadolinium
based *contrast agents*.

See *Gd-DOTA*.

Double balanced mixer

Part of the MRI system that produces an amplitude modified
RF waveform suitable for *slice selection*, by combining the
RF signal with an audio-frequency (AF) waveform.

See also *ADC* and *DAC*.

Double donut

Name for a specific design of magnet with a vertical rather
than horizontal field which can be used as an *open scanner*.

Double inversion recovery

See *black blood preparation*.

Double oblique

Images which are acquired in a non-orthogonal or oblique
plane and also angled in a second additional axis.

Double-tuned

See *dual-tuned*.

Doublet

The appearance of an MRS resonance, which is split into two closely spaced peaks due to *J-coupling*. Examples include *lactate* and *alanine*.

Draining vein

A problem associated with the *BOLD* effect, where the signal response is actually reflecting changes in veins. This results in a spatial shift relative to the true neuronal activation by a few mm.

See also *fMRI*.

References

Turner R. How much cortex can a vein drain? Downstream dilution of activation-related cerebral blood oxygenation changes. Neuroimage. 2002;16:1062–1067

DRESS

Abbreviation for Depth REsolved Surface coil Spectroscopy. The simplest MRS technique involving a 90° excitation pulse used to acquire signal from a cylindrical volume directly underneath a *surface coil*. It is only useful if the tissue being examined is fairly homogenous.

DRIVE

A Philips DRIVEn equilibrium sequence.
See also *driven equilibrium*.

Driven equilibrium

A specific type of MRI pulse sequence where a negative 90° RF pulse is used to force the T_1 relaxation and thereby shorten repetition times. It is principally used to maintain high fluid signal in reduced scan times. Examples include FRFSE (GE), RESTORE (Siemens), DRIVE (Philips) and T2 Plus (Toshiba).

DSA

Abbreviation for Digital Subtraction Angiography. Interventional Radiology technique used to image blood vessels whereby an X-ray is taken with a contrast medium and a pre-contrast image is subtracted to improve visualization. MR Angiography is increasingly used as a less invasive alternative.

DSC

Abbreviation for Dynamic Susceptibility Contrast.
   See also *perfusion imaging*.

DSI

Abbreviation for Diffusion Spectrum Imaging. A method of visualizing fiber tracts that is more accurate than *DTI* in cases of fiber-crossings and intersections.

DSV

Abbreviation for the Diameter of a Spherical Volume. This is a term used to quantify the B_0 homogeneity of a scanner over a given distance. It refers to a volume centered about the *isocenter*, within which changes in the magnetic field should not exceed the stated level. For example, a typical value of "<1 ppm 40 cm DSV," means the field should change by less than 1 Hz per million Hz in any 20 cm direction from the isocenter. For an *open scanner* the corresponding value may be as much as 5 ppm.
   See also B_0 *inhomogeneity*.

DTI

Abbreviation for Diffusion Tensor Imaging. A DWI technique in which at least six diffusion weighted images with different gradient combinations must be acquired to permit the calculation of the diffusion *tensor* (although as many as 55 are now used). By determining the tensor the true 3D nature of the diffusion process can be realized. It is a rotationally invariant measurement (unlike *ADC*), i.e., the values are not governed by the orientation of the structure in relation to the magnetic field.

The diffusion tensor is a symmetric 3×3 matrix:

$$\underline{D} = \begin{bmatrix} D_{xx} & D_{xy} & D_{xz} \\ D_{xy} & D_{yy} & D_{yz} \\ D_{xz} & D_{yz} & D_{zz} \end{bmatrix}$$

Its diagonal elements (D_{xx}, D_{yy}, D_{zz}) correspond to diffusion along three orthogonal axes. The off-diagonal elements relate diffusion between these axes. When these off-diagonal elements are zero, the tensor is said to be diagonalised in order to obtain three *eigenvalues* and eigenvectors which describe the diffusion orientation. The eigenvector with the largest eigenvalue represents the preferred or principal direction of diffusion.

The tensor can be displayed as a 2D image in a number of ways e.g., using a *diffusion ellipsoid* or *colored orientation map*. Alternatively, the principal eigenvector can be used to trace diffusion pathways between connected voxels. This is often used in the brain to visualize white matter tracts and this is termed *tractography*.

References

Arfanakis K, et al. Diffusion tensor MRI in temporal lobe epilepsy. Magn Reson Imaging. 2002;20:511–519
See also *fractional anisotropy*

Dual echo

A specific instance of a multiple echo sequence (e.g., FSE) where two separate images are produced. It is useful for obtaining images of different contrasts, for example a *proton density weighted* image from the early echo time and a T_2 weighted image at the later echo.

Dual slice

Abbreviated to DS. The name of a *simultaneous excitation* sequence from Hitachi.

Dual tune

The ability of an *RF coil* which can be set to the *resonant frequency* of more than one nuclei. Usually, this consists of using proton to provide imaging and localisation and a second non-proton nucleus for MRS. The associated hardware is designated as broad-band to accommodate the required frequency range.

DUFIS

Acronym for DANTE UltraFast Imaging Sequence. A single-shot *burst imaging* method using a *DANTE* RF pulse train with a 180° pulse to refocus a series of spin-echoes.

Dummy

Description a pulse sequence acquisition where no data is recorded. Referred to as DDA on GE scanners (Dummy or Discarded Data Acquisition). An example of its use is in *single-shot* sequences (e.g., fMRI) which allows signal equilibrium to be established.

Duty cycle

The percentage of the repetition time (TR) when the imaging *gradient* is operating at the maximum amplitude. It is an indication of how gradient-intensive a sequence is. For example, in a spin-echo sequence this may be around 10%, but increases to 50% for *EPI*.

DVT imaging

Abbreviation for Deep Vein Thrombosis imaging. Imaging of blood clots due to the resulting T_1 shortening effect, which produces a bright signal on T_1-weighted images.

Dwell time

The time at the beginning of the *FID* during which no signal is recorded due to practical constraints.

DWI

Abbreviation for Diffusion Weighted Imaging. The imaging sequence is sensitized to motion on a molecular level by using a bipolar gradient scheme with very high amplitudes (see *Stejskal-Tanner*). It is of clinical use in *stroke* as ischemic cell swelling reduces the diffusion of water. These changes can be seen much earlier with DWI compared to conventional imaging (Fig. 23).

See also *diffusion*, *ADC*, *ADC map* and *DTI*.

References

Schaefer PW, Grant PE, Gonzalez RG. Diffusion-weighted MR imaging of the brain. Radiology. 2000;217:331–345

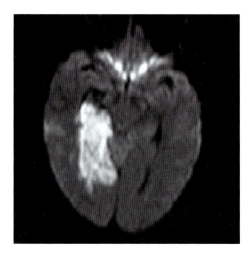

FIGURE 23   A *DWI* brain image with b-factor = 1,000 s mm^{-2} in a patient following a stroke. The ischemic region is clearly visible as high signal indicating restricted diffusion. Liney G. MRI in clinical practice. London: Springer; 2006, p. 66

DWIBS

Acronym for the Philips technique of Diffusion Weighted Imaging with Body background Suppression. This is the use of *DWI* as a *whole-body screening* technique (Fig. 24).

Dynamic

The repeated acquisition of images at the same slice location. Examples of this include *dynamic contrast enhancement* or studying physiological motion e.g., in cardiac MRI.

Dynamic contrast enhancement

Commonly abbreviated to DCE. The specific use of a *dynamic* acquisition following the administration of a *contrast agent* in

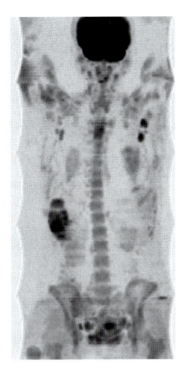

Figure 24 Example of a *DWIBS* type acquisition used as a screening tool to detect axillary lymph node spread in this breast tumor patient

order to study the time dependent characteristics of tissue uptake and wash-out. This can be particularly useful in distinguishing between benign and malignant tumors. Images may be viewed in a *cine* loop or measurements from regions-of-interest can be analyzed graphically to produce a *signal-time curve*. Alternatively, calculations can be made on a pixel-by-pixel basis to produce a single *parameter map* at each slice location. Examples of this vary from simple empirical measurements of maximum enhancement to more complicated information from *pharmacokinetic modeling* (Fig. 25).

See also *Type I,II,III*

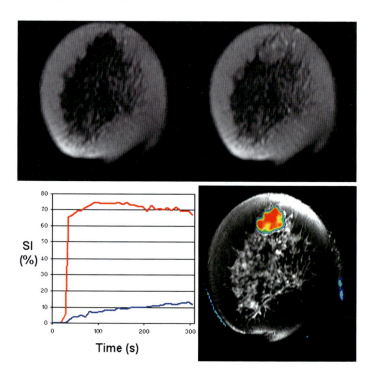

Figure 25 A *dynamic contrast enhancement* study in the breast (*top*). Comparison of the first image in the time series on the left with one acquired 20 s later on the right reveals a suspicious area of enhancement on the *bottom left*, a plot of signal enhancement against time for the tumor is shown in red and for a normal region in blue. On the *bottom right*, the enhancement is determined on pixel-by-pixel basis and shown as a color map overlaid onto a high resolution fat suppressed image. Liney G. MRI in clinical practice. London: Springer; 2006, p. 80, 81

Dynamic nuclear polarization

A particular type of *hyperpolarisation* technique used to improve the MRI signal of a low sensitivity nucleus (e.g., ^{13}C).

At fairly low temperatures and high fields (e.g., 1 K and 3.0 T) electrons are highly polarized and this polarization is transferred to the nuclei using microwaves.

See also *parahydrogen-induced polarization.*

Dynamic susceptibility contrast

See *perfusion imaging.*

E

eADC

Abbreviation for *exponential ADC*. Note the lowercase "e" convention.

Earth's magnetic field

The magnetic field experienced on the Earth's surface due to electrical currents in the iron of the outer core. It acts as a *dipole* with an approximate 11° difference between the magnetic and geographic poles. The strength of the field varies from approximately 0.3 G at the equator to 0.7 Gauss at the poles.

Earth's field MRI

Also known as Earth's field NMR or EFNMR. This refers to the concept of using the extremely low strength geomagnetic field to produce MR spectroscopy or imaging. The absence of any internally produced static field means that systems can be made extremely lightweight and portable. They are useful for teaching aids and monitoring changes in the Earth's magnetic field. Images typically take several hours to acquire due to the low signal.

ECG

Abbreviation for ElectroCardioGraph (also sometimes written as EKG). The ECG is characterized by the *PQRST wave*.
    See also *ECG gating*.

ECG gating

Specific type of image *gating* or triggering based on the ECG signal. Electrodes placed across the chest measure changes in voltage during the cardiac cycle.

See also *PQRST wave*, *vectorcardiograph* and *peripheral pulse gating*.

Echo modulation

The phenomenon exhibited by coupled spins in multiple pulse sequences which causes signal decay to be modulated. General signal intensity equations relate to uncoupled spins only. So-called *AX systems* are only weakly coupled but the signal response for strongly coupled spins (*AB systems*) demonstrates a greater modulation of signal amplitude on top of normal T_2 decay. In *citrate* for example there is a fast phase change of the outer two resonances which has a period of approximately 135 ms. The exact nature of the signal changes depends on the sequence, for example modulations are more pronounced with *PRESS* than with *STEAM*. These signal characteristics also vary with field strength.

Echo planar imaging

See *EPI*.

Echo spacing

The interval between each successive echo in a multiple echo train sequence e.g., FSE or EPI. Also known as inter echo time, inter echo spacing (IES) or echo train internal (ETI).

Echo time

See *TE*.

Echo train

Referring to a series of closely spaced signal echoes produced within a single repetition time (TR).

Echo train length

Abbreviated to ETL, it is equal to the number of echoes in an echo train. If these echoes are separately phase encoded (see *FSE*), then the scan time is reduced by a factor equal to the phase encoding matrix divided by the ETL (e.g., for ETL = 32 and 256 matrix the scan is 8 (=256/32) times faster).

ED

Annotation on a *DICOM* image meaning Extended Dynamic range.

   See also *EDR*.

Eddy currents

The undesirable result of the rapidly changing magnetic fields in the gradient coils. These induce oscillating currents which in turn create their own magnetic fields in the *cryostat* and adjacent conductors. As a result, the linearity of the gradient is altered leading to image distortion which has to be compensated by using *pre-emphasis* or gradient *shielding*.

Edge enhancement

1. Characteristic increase in signal at the edges of tissue due to motion between successive *dynamic contrast enhancement* scans. The pixels at the boundary move between tissue and low signal in the background thereby appearing to

enhance on subtracted images or associated parameter maps. This may be remedied by restricting the movement of anatomy or using *motion correction*.
2. Also may be used to describe preferential contrast uptake at the periphery of some tumors (see *rim enhancement*).

EDR

Abbreviation for Extended Dynamic Range. This is a (GE) scanner setting, which increases the dynamic range of the receiver amplifier. Failure to accommodate the signal range may result in *over-ranging* and produce a *halo artifact*.

EEG

Abbreviation for ElectroEncephaloGraphy. The Measurement of electrical currents in the brain in order to examine brain function. The technique has poor spatial resolution but very high temporal resolution compared to *fMRI*.
  See also *MEG*.

Effective TE

The time of the central echo in the *echo train* of a fast spin-echo sequence. The image contrast is determined by this effective value although multiple echoes at different TEs are used.

Efficiency

Defined as the signal-to-noise ratio (see *SNR*) of an image divided by the square root of the acquisition time. This allows a comparison to be made between different sequences with different imaging times.

Eigenvalues

The coefficients of the (diagonalised) diffusion tensor (see *DTI*), which give the magnitude of diffusion along each of three mutually orthogonal directions. These directions are given by the corresponding three eigenvectors.

See also *fractional anisotropy*.

Einthoven's triangle

The equilateral triangular positioning of the three electrodes used in *ECG gating*.

Ejection fraction

A calculation used to assess cardiac function in *cardiac MRI*. It is defined as a percentage (EF) from:

$$EF = 100 \times (EDV - ESV)/EDV$$

where EDV and ESV are the End Diastolic Volume and End Systolic Volume respectively as defined by manually drawn regions-of-interest from appropriate MR images.

Elastogram

A parameter map produced from an elastography study (see *MRE*). It displays the stiffness or strain of tissue with tumors showing between 5 and 28 times larger values compared to normal tissue.

Elastography

See *MRE*.

Electron

A subatomic particle that exists in orbits around the nucleus. It has a charge equal to 1.602×10^{-19} C (the unit of elementary charge) and a mass of 9.109×10^{-31} kg.

Electron shielding

See *shielding constant*.
    See also *chemical shift*.

Electron spin resonance

Abbreviated to ESR. An alternative term for electron paramagnetic resonance (see *EPR*).

Elliptic centric k-space filling

Type of *centric k-space filling* used in 3D imaging, which also takes into account the order of the phase encoding steps in the third dimension or "slice" direction. It is used in 3D *MRA* to improve the temporal efficiency of the sequence. Known as Elliptical scanning on Siemens systems.

Elongatedness

A measure used to describe the degree of elongation of a shape or region. It is related to the number of iterations of a thinning algorithm needed to reduce the border down to a minimally connected stroke, with long thin shapes having the smallest values.
    See also *morphological descriptors*.

Endogenous contrast

Referring to the variations of image contrast due to inherent tissue differences e.g., due to diffusion effects relaxation times etc. The opposite of *exogenous contrast*.

Endorectal coil

An RF *surface coil* consisting of coil loop inside either an inflatable balloon or rigid probe and inserted into the vagina or rectum. Inflatable coils tend to reduce organ movement but at high field, air-inflated coils are not used due to the increased *susceptibility artifact*. Other filling materials have been used at high field e.g., *perflurocarbon*.

These coils are particularly prone to signal flare i.e., extremely bright signal close to the surface which drops off rapidly further away from the coil (Fig. 26).

See also *coil uniformity correction*.

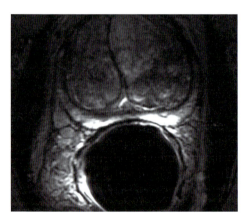

FIGURE 26 An *endorectal coil* image of the prostate displaying its characteristic signal flare. Liney G. MRI in clinical practice. London: Springer; 2006, p. 94

Endorem

Commercial name of an iron-based contrast agent developed by AMAG Pharmaceuticals and Guerbet. It is taken up in the normal liver thereby improving the conspicuity of liver lesions. It consists of a *dextran*-coated ferumoxide and has also been referred to as AMI-25 and Feridex.

See also *liver-specific contrast agents*.

Enhancement

An increase in signal intensity (usually) caused by the administration of *contrast agents*. It may also refer to increasing the signal of low sensitivity nuclei by the process of *hyperpolarisation*.

Enhancement rate

A measurement taken from a *signal-time curve* used to display *dynamic contrast enhancement* data. It is a measure of how fast the contrast is taken up by the tissue and is equal to the maximum change divided by the time interval i.e., the steepest gradient in the curve.

See also *MITR*.

Enteral agents

Type of *contrast agents* that are administered either orally or rectally.

See also *oral contrast agents*.

Entry-slice phenomenon

Synonym for *in-flow enhancement*.

EPI

Abbreviation for Echo Planar Imaging. An ultra-fast imaging sequence first proposed by P. Mansfield in 1977, in which combinations of the gradients are used to traverse *k-space* as fast as possible. The sequence can be utilized as either *single-shot* or *multi-shot*. The imaging matrix size is usually limited to between 64 and 128. It is used whenever imaging speed is more important than quality e.g., pediatrics, fMRI. Commonly *blipped EPI* is performed but both *constant EPI* and *spiral EPI* sequences are also used. The sequence is inherently noisy (see *acoustic noise*).

In EPI the high receiver bandwidth ensures *chemical shift artifact* in the frequency direction is negligible. However, the repeated application of phase encoding gradients within one shot causes phase differences between fat and water to accumulate leading to a water-fat shift of tens of pixels in the phase direction.

EPI is also prone to geometric distortions caused by gradient non-linearities. This is particularly prominent in areas of inherent B_0 *inhomogeneity* e.g., frontal and temporal lobes. The nature of the gradient switching means EPI images also suffer from *Nyquist ghosting*. Examples of EPI are shown in Figs. 1 and 62 (Fig. 27).

References

Mansfield P. Real time echo planar imaging by NMR. Br Med Bull. 1984;40:187–190

EPISTAR

Type of *arterial spin labeling* sequence employing saturation as opposed to inversion as a labeling method. It is an acronym of EPI-Signal Tagging with Alternating Radiofrequency.

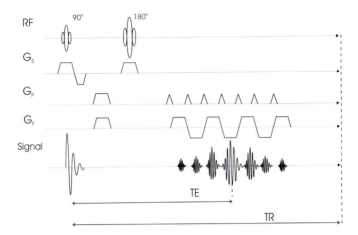

FIGURE 27 Pulse sequence diagram for the *EPI* sequence. G_S, G_P and G_F represent the gradients for the slice selection, phase encoding and frequency encoding respectively. The gradients are played out in such a way as to acquire all the k-space data as quickly as possible. EPI can be thought of as a fast read-out module with image contrast coming from (in this case) a spin-echo sequence. Liney G. MRI in clinical practice. London: Springer; 2006, p. 19

EPI factor

The number of times (or shots) the EPI sequence has to be run in order to acquire the image data.

EPIC

The *pulse programming* language on GE systems.

EPR

Abbreviation for Electron Paramagnetic Resonance. Analogous to the nuclear magnetic resonance phenomenon but observed in unpaired electrons (generally as free radicals). Due to the much smaller mass of the electron, weaker magnetic fields and higher frequencies are used compared with MRI (e.g., 0.3 T and 10 GHz).

Ernst angle

The optimal flip angle needed to produce the maximum signal when a reduced TR ($TR \ll T_1$) is used in *gradient echo* imaging. It is related to both TR and T_1 by:

$$Cos\ \alpha_E = \exp\left(-TR / T_1\right)$$

For $TR \gg T_1$ the optimal flip angle becomes 90°, as in the case of a spin-echo sequence.

See also *partial flip*.

ETL

Abbreviation for *Echo Train Length*.

Eurospin test objects

A commonly used set of test objects (Diagnostic Sonar Ltd) each with a specific design and purpose. Their name and purpose are given below:

TO1 = A *floodfill phantom*
TO2 = A *geometric distortion* and slice *profile phantom*
TO3 = A phantom for assessing *slice warp* and position
TO4 = A spatial *resolution phantom*
TO5 = A set of *gel phantoms* for contrast and relaxation time
    measurements

References

Lerski RA, de Certaines JD. Performance assessment and quality control in MRI by Eurospin test objects and protocols. Magn Reson Imaging. 1993;11(6):817–833

Even echo rephasing

Referring to the phenomenon where, due to the quadratic nature of phase loss by spins moving in the presence of a gradient, signal at evenly spaced echoes becomes re-phased. Phase loss of moving spins is given by:

$$\varphi = \tfrac{1}{2} \gamma \, Gvt^2$$

where ϕ is phase, G, gradient strength, v, velocity of motion, and t, the time interval under consideration.

See also *odd-echo dephasing*.

Event related

Type of *fMRI* experiment where the stimuli are randomly presented and are usually of shorter duration then those used in a *box car* experiment.

Excitation pulse

A radio-frequency (RF) pulse used to transmit the B_1 field in order to turn the net magnetization towards the receiver coil in the *transverse plane* for detection. In normal circumstances the optimum signal is achieved with a 90° (or $\pi/2$) pulse.

See also *refocusing pulse*.

Exogenous contrast

Referring to any externally administered contrast agent (usually intravenously) which is given to improve the differentiation of tissues within the image.

See also *endogenous contrast*.

Exponential

A function that increases or decreases at a rate equal to its current value. The derivative of an exponential function is the value of the function itself. It can be further defined as:

$$e^x = 1 + x + x^2 / 2! + x^3 / 3! + \ldots$$

Exponential functions appear frequently in MRI as they describe *relaxation* mechanisms (see *Bloch equations*).

The *Fourier transformation* of an exponential is a *Lorentzian shape*.

Exponential ADC

A diffusion weighted image (see *DWI*) where the effect of T_2 *shine through* has been removed. It is usually written as eADC. The image retains the same contrast as a normal diffusion weighted image (i.e., signal decrease with high ADC).

Exposure limits

See *safety limits*.

EXPRESS

Picker's single-shot FSE sequence.

Extended dynamic range

See EDR.

External interference shield

A further set of coil windings outside of the *shielding* windings, through which current flows to counteract the effects of large moving metal objects (e.g., cars) in the vicinity of the scanner.

See B_0 *homogeneity* and *proximity limits*.

Extracellular agents

The most common type of MRI contrast agent currently in use. These diffuse freely into non-vascular extracellular space thereby limiting their use as a *blood-pool agent*.

F

FA

Abbreviation for *Fractional Anisotropy*.

FACT

Acronym for the *tractography* algorithm called Fiber Assignment by means of Continuous Tracking. This method uses a minimum threshold of *fractional anisotropy* together with a maximum trajectory angle in order to map out connected fibers.

FADE

Acronym for the Fast Acquisition with Dual Echo sequence. A Picker sequence similar to *DESS*.

FAIR

Type of *arterial spin labeling* sequence which is an acronym of Flow-sensitive Alternative Inversion Recovery. A non-selective inversion pulse excites the whole volume and an image slice is recorded. Subsequently a selective inversion is performed on the imaging slice only to magnetically label spins for perfusion measurement.

FAISE

Acronym for Fast Acquisition Interleaved Spin Echo. Name for a sequence that is similar to *RARE*, *FSE* etc.

Fall time

Opposite of the *rise time* of a gradient waveform.

FAME

Acronym for FAst Multi Echo sequence. Equivalent to the *FSE* sequence.

Faraday cage

The copper lining within the walls, ceiling and floor of the scan room to prevent extraneous radio-frequency sources from entering the scanner, which would otherwise cause an *RF artifact*. The scan room door must be closed to maintain the integrity of the cage and usually the scanner notifies the user if the door is left open prior to scanning. The window between the scan room and control room also contains a copper mesh within it (Fig. 28).

See also *wave guides*.

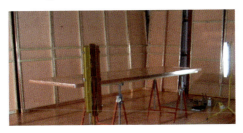

FIGURE 28 Photo showing the construction of the *faraday cage* prior to the installation of a new scanner

Faraday's law

Law of physics which describes the emf (electromotive force or voltage) induced in a conductor when surrounded by a changing magnetic field. This is the basis of the *eddy currents* caused by the action of the gradient coils. The emf (ε) is proportional to the rate of change of the magnetic *flux* (φ):

$$\varepsilon = -\frac{\partial \phi}{\partial t}$$

The negative sign is due to *Lenz's law*.

FASE

Acronym for Fast Advanced Spin-Echo. A single-shot FSE sequence from Toshiba.

FAST

Acronym for Fourier Acquired STeady state. This sequence is also seen prefixed with RF (RF spoiled) or RAM (Rapidly Acquired Magnetization).

See also *Spoiling*.

FASTCARD

A *cine* cardiac imaging sequence from GE.

See also *cardiac MRI.*

Fast Fourier transform

Abbreviated to FFT. This is an efficient computer algorithm of the discrete *Fourier transformation* used in the reconstruction of MRI. A common FFT is the Cooley–Tukey algorithm.

References

Brigham EO. The fast Fourier transform and its applications. Englewood Cliffs: Prentice-Hall; 1988. ISBN 0133075052

Fast gradient echo

Generic term for gradient echo sequences which use *spoiling*. See also *FSPGR.*

Fast IR

Fast Inversion Recovery. An FSE sequence that is preceded with an *inversion recovery* pulse.

Fast recovery FSE

A *driven equilibrium* sequence from GE.

Fast spin echo

See *FSE.*

Fat

The second most dominant contribution to the proton MR signal. The fat signal is made up of different *lipid* resonances, which may need suppressing to obtain MR spectra in certain areas of the body (e.g., near the scalp, or in breast). At 1.5 T the main fat resonance is 220 Hz from water or at 1.3 ppm.

See also *fat-water in-phase, fat suppression* and *chemical shift artifact.*

Fat fraction

Quantification of the relative amount of fat signal in a given voxel. It may be expressed as the fat-to-water ratio (FWR) or as the fat fraction (FF) which is equal to the fat signal divided by the total (water+fat) signal. Measurements are made with either MR spectroscopy, or fat and water-only imaging, with the latter having the advantage of improved resolution albeit only the main *lipid* signal is usually recorded. MRS offers the potential to quantify unsaturated and saturated fat fractions which has been shown to be important in *bone imaging*.

Fat only image

An image based on signal from the fat resonance only and not the combined water and fat signal as in routine imaging. This is produced from the subtraction of an *in-phase image* and *out-of-phase image* in sequences such as *DIXON* (Fig. 29).

See also *chemical shift* (*"of the second kind"*) and *fat-water in-phase*.

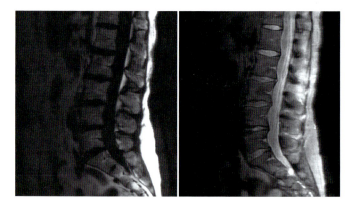

FIGURE 29 A *fat-only image* (*left*) in the lumbar spine created by the subtraction of in-phase and out-of-phase images. This image highlights the fat content in bone marrow and can be compared to the corresponding water only image (*right*) created from the summation of in and out-of-phase images

Fat saturation

Also referred to as fat sat. This is a method of *fat suppression* that utilizes a narrow RF pulse (see *CHESS*).

Fat suppression

Referring to one of the many methods of eliminating the contribution of the fat signal in the image. Each technique takes advantage of the differences between fat and water in terms of chemical shift, phase or relaxation time. Common techniques include *CHESS*, *STIR*, *Dixon* and *SPIR* (Fig. 30).

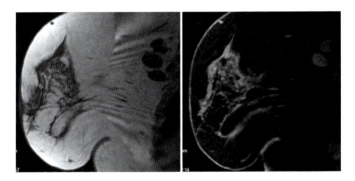

FIGURE 30 (*Left*) A T_1-weighted breast image and (*right*) the same image with *fat suppression* using a fat saturation (CHESS) pulse

Fat-water in-phase

Referring to the use of particular echo times so that the fat and water signals are acquired in-phase. The echo time is dependent on field strength. The frequency difference between fat and water is equal to 220 Hz at 1.5 T, meaning the signals are in-phase every 1/220 s. The in-phase values are therefore given by even multiples of 2.3 ms (i.e., 4.6, 9.2...) and odd multiples give the out of phase condition (i.e., 2.3,

6.9…). At 3.0 T this value becomes 1.2 ms (i.e., 2.4, 4.8…in-phase and 1.2, 3.6…out of phase). Most scanners allow the user to set the echo time to be in or out of phase automatically (Fig. 31).

See also *chemical shift ("of the second kind")* and *OOPS*.

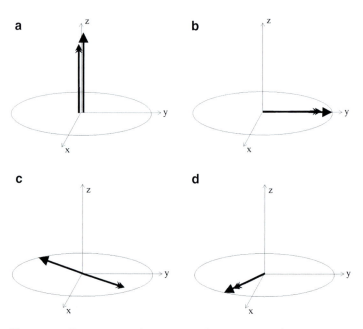

FIGURE 31 *Fat-water in-phase*. Precession of the fat (*double arrow head*) and water spins following an RF excitation pulse (**a, b**). The fat and water signals cycle between being exactly (**c**) out of phase or (**d**) in phase at certain echo times

FATE

Acronym for FAst Turbo Echo.

FatSep

Name of the *DIXON* type fat separation technique used on Hitachi systems.

FBI

Abbreviation for Fresh Blood Imaging. A non-contrast enhanced MRA sequence from Toshiba. Other similar sequences include InHance (GE), TRANCE (Philips), NATIVE (Siemens), and VASC (Hitachi).

FC

Annotation on a *DICOM* image meaning Flow Compensation.

FE

Abbreviation of Field-Echo, an old term for gradient-echo.

FEDIF

Abbreviation of Field-Echo DIFFerence. A gradient echo sequence with the echo time set so that fat and water are out of phase.

See *Chemical shift ("of the second kind")* and *fat-water in-phase*

Feet first entry

Referring to the patient position on the bed when imaging the lower part of the body. This enables the head to be nearer to the outside of the scanner making it less claustrophobic.

See also *head first entry*.

Fermi filter

Common filter used in *apodisation*. Its characteristic shape is defined by:

$$F(x) = \frac{1}{\left(e^{(x-D)/T} + 1\right)}$$

where D and T are known as the Fermi diameter and transmission width.

Ferridex

Commercial name for one of the *liver-specific contrast agents*, and is also known as *Endorem*.

Ferrogaurd

Commercial name of a wall-mounted or free-standing patient screening device that is sensitive to ferromagnetic material without detecting other metallic material that is MR safe.

Ferromagnetic

Property of material with an extremely high positive susceptibility (e.g., iron). Magnetic field domains are induced within a ferromagnetic object when it is brought close to the scanner turning it into a *projectile*. Patients are screened for such objects or implants prior to examination.

See also *paramagnetic* and *diamagnetic*.

Ferucarbotran

The generic name for the contrast agent *Resovist*.

Ferumoxtran

The generic name for the contrast agents *Endorem* and *Sinerem*.

FESUM

Abbreviation of Field-Echo SUMmation. A gradient echo sequence with the echo time set so that fat and water are in phase.

See also *chemical shift ("of the second kind")* and *fat-water in-phase*

FFT

Abbreviation for *Fast Fourier Transform*.

FFT scale

Abbreviation for Fast Fourier Transform scale. A system setting on Siemens scanners, controlling the receiver gain.

See also *pre-scan*.

FGRET

A GE sequence, from the abbreviation of Fast GRadient echo-Echo Train. Combines a gradient echo with an EPI readout, to provide a high temporal resolution scan (typically 1–2 s). Predominantly used for rapid cardiac visualization.

Fiber tracking

See *tractography*.

FID

Acronym for Free Induction Decay. The signal produced immediately following an excitation pulse, characterized by an initial peak and a rapid decay due to T_2^* effects. The term induction arises from the current, which is induced in a coil by the rotating magnetization. A FID is shown in Fig. 83.

FID artifact

A broken line of signal that occurs at the center of the image along the frequency encoding direction i.e., at zero phase encoding. This can be easily misinterpreted as an *RF artifact* although it is in the other direction. The artifact is due to the *FID* signal being detected with the echo. Since the FID signal is not phase encoded the artifact is not dispersed along the phase encoding direction and appears as a single line at the center. It arises due to a combination of poor B_1 homogeneity and slice profile together with insufficient spoiler gradients.

Field decay

Referring to the loss of the B_0 magnetic field due to imperfections in the *superconductor* e.g., at the soldered joins. It typically accounts for 5–10 G loss of field per annum. In a *permanent magnet* and *resistive magnet*, factors such as aging, temperature and power supply are also important.

Field-of-view

More commonly known by the abbreviation FOV. This is the area being imaged and may be symmetrical or rectangular. The FOV is related to the amplitude of the phase (G_p) and frequency (G_F) gradients as follows:

$$\gamma G_F = BW / FOV$$
$$\gamma G_p t_p = 0.5 N_p / FOV$$

where BW, N_p and t_p are the receiver bandwidth, phase encoding matrix and the duration of the phase encoding gradient respectively.

See also *rectangular FOV* and *off-center FOV*.

Field stability

The expected drift in the *center frequency* of the system with time. Typically the center frequency should vary by <0.1 ppm h^{-1}.

FIESTA

Acronym for Fast Imaging Employing Steady sTATe. A true refocused steady-state free precession sequence. This sequence is useful in increasing the edge effect at tissue interfaces.

See also *true FISP*.

Filling factor

The relationship between the size of the RF coil and the volume of tissue within the coil. The greater the percentage of the coil volume being filled by the tissue the better the *SNR*.

See also *loading*.

Filter

The utilization of some time or frequency domain filter to improve some property of the image usually with a trade-off in some other characteristic. For example the *SNR* may be improved at the expense of spatial resolution. Some scanners apply filters by default prior to image display and care needs to be taken to turn these off prior to any *quality assurance* measurements being made.

See also *apodisation*.

Filtered back projection

Image reconstruction method used in *projection reconstruction* where a series of image profiles are filtered prior to back projection in order to improve the final image. Used in CT and nuclear medicine (but no longer in MRI).

Finger tapping

A commonly used functional MRI *paradigm*. This involves getting the patient to move their fingers and thumbs together repeatedly to elicit a response in the opposite primary motor area of the brain.

See also *inverse lateralisation*

FIR

Abbreviation for Fast Inversion Recovery (see *Fast IR*).

First pass

Referring to the first time the contrast agent arrives from the site of injection to the imaging site. Subsequent signal changes are due to the recirculation of blood. In myocardial perfusion studies this is extremely fast requiring high temporal resolution imaging.

FISP

Acronym for Fast Imaging with Steady state Precession. A Siemens *steady-state* sequence using rewinding gradients in the phase encoding direction only.

See also *bFFE*.

Five gauss line

The proximity limit around the scanner within which entry for patients with pacemakers is precluded. Five gauss is equivalent to 0.5 mT.

See also *fringe field*.

FLAG

Acronym for FLow Adjusted Gradients.

See also *flow compensation*.

FLAIR

Acronym for FLuid Attenuated Inversion Recovery. Name of GE's *long tau inversion recovery* sequence.

FLARE

1. Acronym for Fast Low Angle Recalled Echo. A sequence similar to *FLASH*.
2. Referring to the appearance of extremely bright tissue signal immediately next to a *surface coil* (see Figs. 14 and 26).

FLASE

Acronym for Fast Large Angle Spin Echo.

FLASH

A Siemens spoiled gradient echo sequence which is an acronym from Fast Low Angle Snap sHot. This is a rapid gradient echo sequence using a small flip angle and short TR. In *Turbo FLASH* the TR is so short that T_1 contrast is maintained by using an inversion pulse. The GE equivalent to this is the *FSPGR* sequence.

Flashing artifact

Bright signal seen in the first cardiac gated image following the R wave due to T_1 relaxation, which has occurred in the non-imaged part of the cycle. It can be avoided by acquiring *dummy* data immediately after the R wave.

Flip angle

The resulting orientation, α degrees, of the net magnetization with respect to the B_0 field, following the application of an RF *excitation pulse*. It is given by:

$$\alpha = \gamma B_1 t$$

where B_1 and t is the strength and duration of the RF pulse respectively, and γ is the *gyromagnetic ratio*. The flip angle is also related to the *SAR*.

Floodfill phantom

A homogenous phantom designed to enable signal-to-noise ratio (*SNR*) and *uniformity* measurements to be taken. Usually several different sizes are provided for use with different RF coils and these can be cylinders or spheres. An example is shown on the left of Fig. 66.

See also *quality assurance*.

Flow artifacts

Image artifacts specifically caused by flowing spins for example due to vascular flow. Commonly observed as *ghosting* in the phase encoding direction, which is most apparent when the blood flow is perpendicular to the imaging plane. Additionally an apparent lateral displacement of vessels may occur in *even-echo rephasing*, where the vessel is in the imaging plane but has an oblique orientation to the frequency encoding direction.

Flow compensation

Imaging technique incorporating additional gradients (sometimes called FLAG or FLow Adjusted Gradients) to reduce intravoxel dephasing. This improves the uniformity of blood signal and reduces CSF flow effects etc. It is denoted on a *DICOM* image as FC.

See also *gradient-moment nulling*.

Flow phenomena

Referring to the MRI effects of flowing blood which can result in either an increase or decrease of signal intensity. Flow can be characterized as laminar, were the flow has a parabolic profile with the highest velocities at the center of the vessel, or turbulent where the profile is flat towards the center. The onset of turbulent flow is predicted from the *Reynolds number*. *In-flow enhancement* causes flowing blood to appear bright. Signal voids are caused by *high velocity signal loss* and also dephasing due to motion along a gradient (see *phase contrast*).

Flow-related enhancement

See *In-flow enhancement*.

Flow void

Signal loss due to the motion of (usually) blood and taken advantage of in *black blood* angiography.

Fluorine

The MR visible isotope of fluorine is ^{19}F, which has the second highest sensitivity of all nuclei. Virtually absent in the human body, it is extremely useful in monitoring fluorinated drugs (e.g., 5FU or gemcitabin in chemotherapy) as there is no background signal. The gas itself may be imaged in *lung MRI* although this is not currently for human use.

MR properties of ^{19}F:

Spin quantum number = 1/2
Sensitivity = 0.8300
Natural abundance = 100.00%
Gyromagnetic ratio = 40.05 MHz T^{-1}.

Fluoroptic thermometer

A type of MR compatible thermometer that is often used to measure temperature changes due to *RF heating* effects. The device works by emitting a red light to a phosphor probe causing infrared fluorescence and the time taken for this to decay indicates the local temperature.

Fluorotrigger

GE's implementation of *bolus tracking*.

FLUTE

Acronym for FLUoro TriggEred MRA. Name for the *bolus tracking* sequence on Hitachi systems.

Flux

The lines of force associated with a magnetic field; the number per unit area is known as the flux density.

fMRI

Abbreviation for Functional MRI. The "f" is always written in lower-case by convention. A non-invasive method of studying brain function. The most commonly used technique relies on *BOLD* contrast. It permits the visualization of active areas of the brain due to the local response in blood flow. fMRI is used generally in the research of cognition but it is also being increasingly used for *surgical planning* and *radiotherapy planning* in order to avoid damage to these functional areas.

The procedure involves rapidly imaging the patient's brain while they are repeatedly subjected to a specific task or stimulus interspersed with control or rest periods (see *paradigm*). The resulting changes in oxygen fraction produce small signal increases which can be correlated to the timing of the stimulus and subsequently yield an *activation map* (Fig. 32).

References

Gowland P, Francis S, Morris P, Bowtell R. Watching the brain at work. Physics World. 2002;15(12):31–35
See also *Wada test*

Foldover

Alternative term for aliasing or *phase wrap* which is used on Philips systems.

Foldover suppression

See *no phase wrap*.

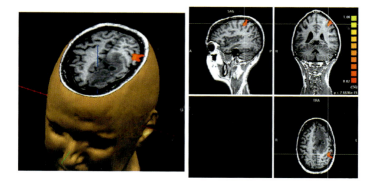

FIGURE 32 Activation maps from an *fMRI* examination of the motor cortex. Images are shown in each orthogonal plane together with a 3D surface rendering. Pixels that significantly correlate with the stimulus paradigm are colored to highlight the area of activation. In this case a right hand task has activated the left motor area close to the tumor and this information can be used in surgery to prevent damage to the motor cortex

Fonar

The oldest MRI company, producing the first clinical MRI system in 1980. It currently sells a unique upright multi-positional system that allows the patient to be imaged in a variety of positions (so called *positional MRI*). This makes it extremely patient friendly but also allows weight-bearing images to be obtained.

www.fonar.com

Footprint

The siting requirement of the MRI scanner which is determined by the extent of its *fringe field*. This typically may be as small as 35 m^2 for modern magnets with *active shielding*.

Foreign bodies

Referring to any implant or material within the patient which may cause artifacts or safety issues.

See *MR compatible*.

Fourier transformation

A Mathematical algorithm (abbreviated to FT) in which time varying signals can be decomposed into a series of sinusoidal components of varying frequency, phase and amplitude. It is the process by which the recorded MR signal is decoded into an image (see *Fast Fourier Transform*).

The Fourier transform of a time varying signal S(t) is given by:

$$S(t) = a_0 + a_1 \sin(\omega_1 t + \varphi_1) + a_2 \sin(\omega_2 t + \varphi_2) + \ldots$$

Some common Fourier transform pairs are given below:

S(t)	S(ω)
Sinc	rectangular
Sinusoid (sine wave)	delta (a single frequency)
Gaussian	Gaussian
Exponential (or *FID* shape)	Lorentzian
Rectangular	Sinc

Figures 50 and 83 illustrate the use of Fourier transformation in MRI.

See also *sinc shaped*.

Fractional anisotropy

A dimensionless quantity, abbreviated to FA, which is a measure of the directional dependence of diffusion in each image voxel. It is a scalar quantity derived from the diffusion *tensor* and is given by:

$$FA = \sqrt{\frac{\left(\lambda_1 - \lambda_2\right)^2 + (\lambda_2 - \lambda_3)^2 + (\lambda_3 - \lambda_1)^2}{2\left(\lambda_1^2 + \lambda_2^2 + \lambda_3^2\right)}}$$

where $\lambda_1 \dots \lambda_3$ are the *eigenvalues* from the diffusion tensor (see *DTI*).

FA has values ranging from 0 to 1. Zero anisotropy (FA = 0), is equivalent to a perfectly isotropic or spherical diffusion path. FA is equal to 1 when $\lambda_1 >> \lambda_2 = \lambda_3$, which describes a cylindrical diffusion path (see *diffusion ellipsoid*).

FA values in the brain can range from 0.2 to 0.9 depending on the region, while they are around 0.1 in CSF and tumors.

FA values are used in *tractography* algorithms to map out fiber trajectories (see *FACT*).

A similar but less commonly used measure is the *relative anisotropy* (RA) (Fig. 33).

Fractional echo

Alternative name for *partial echo*.

Fractional NEX

Refers to an incomplete acquisition of k-space in the phase encoding direction. It should not be confused with the use of the term *NEX* referring to signal averaging.

See also *partial Fourier*.

Frame of reference

Position from which the behavior of spins is viewed in order to more easily describe the action of the RF pulse. Two commonly used references are the *rotating frame* and the *laboratory frame*.

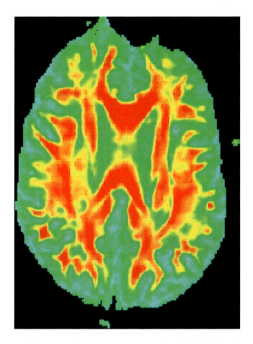

FIGURE 33 A *fractional anisotropy* map in the brain demonstrates the distribution of white matter fibers due to the higher (*red/yellow*) values of FA

Free induction decay

See *FID*.

Free protons

Description of free-flowing water molecules with high *molecular tumbling rate* and a corresponding *short correlation time* (e.g., bladder urine, CSF). This is the opposite of *bound protons*. Other protons may be termed intermediate or structured protons.

Freeze frame

Name of the *time-resolved MRA* sequence from Toshiba.

Frequency

Generally referring to the number of times an event is repeated per unit time. In terms of waves and oscillations it is the number of cycles per second and is measured in Hertz. The reciprocal of frequency is the period.

See also *angular frequency*.

Frequency encoding

The use of a *gradient* to induce linear changes in resonant frequencies, which vary with distance so that the signal may be spatially encoded. Unlike *phase encoding*, encoding with frequency is performed only once at the time of the echo measurement. The frequency encoding gradient will also contain a *dephasing lobe* to ensure no phase loss at the time of the echo. *Chemical shift artifact* is observed in the frequency encoding direction (Fig. 34).

Frequency wrap

Referring to *Aliasing*, which occurs in the frequency encoding direction. This is usually avoided by the use of filters and rapid sampling at the *Nyquist frequency* which is applied by most scanners automatically.

See also *oversampling* and *phase wrap*.

Fresh spins

Description of nuclear spins that have yet to be excited by an RF pulse (see *in-flow enhancement*).

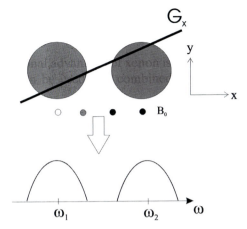

FIGURE 34 Illustration of *frequency encoding*. In this example two circular samples (e.g., from the slice acquired in Fig. 87) are spatially encoded in the x direction by applying an appropriate gradient (G_x). This increases the field strength (denoted by the *darkening circles*) and resonant frequencies of the spins in a linear fashion separating the left and right samples. Phase encoding is then required to spatially discriminate the second (y) dimension. Liney G. MRI in clinical practice. London: Springer; 2006, p. 12

FRFSE

Abbreviation of **Fast Recovery** FSE. A *driven equilibrium* FSE sequence (**Fig. 35**).

Fringe field

The magnetic field produced by the scanner, which extends beyond the scan room (or more specifically outside the imaging volume). It may be reduced by the use of *active shielding*. The fringe field drops off quickly from the magnet and has both axial (z direction) and radial (x,y) components. The axial field is greater than the radial field at any given distance. For

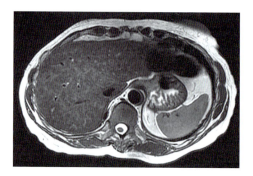

FIGURE 35 A liver image acquired in a single breath-hold of 21 s with the *FRFSE* sequence. Liney G. MRI in clinical practice. London: Springer; 2006, p. 86

a modern (closed bore) scanner it is greater by a factor of approximately 1.6; for example a field of 5 G may be measured at a distance of 2.5 m in the radial direction and 4.0 m in the axial direction.

See also *five gauss line* and *proximity limits*.

FSE

Abbreviation for Fast Spin Echo. An commonly used sequence which consists of multiple 180° refocusing pulses to produce echoes with different phase encoding steps (unlike *multiple spin-echo*). It is used predominantly to produce fast T_2-weighted images. Multiple echoes are used to rapidly obtain an image with an *effective TE* equal to the central echo. The reduced acquisition time is related to the *echo train length*, or ETL, which is typically set to 16 or 32. Excessively long ETLs can cause blurring. FSE-XL, is an enhanced sequence from GE with blurring cancelation. The sequence exists under many different names (e.g., *TSE*) and was originally implemented as *RARE* (Fig. 36).

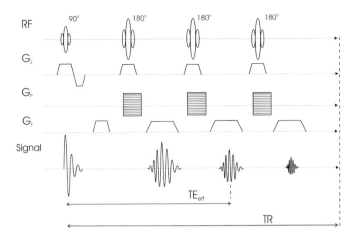

FIGURE 36 Pulse sequence diagram for the *FSE* sequence. G_s, G_p and G_F represent the gradients for the slice selection, phase encoding and frequency encoding respectively. The hatched lines of G_p indicate that this amplitude is varied incrementally. A series of echoes is generated and each one is differently phase encoded so that an image at a single effective echo time (TE_{eff}) is generated much more quickly. Liney G. MRI in clinical practice. London: Springer; 2006, p. 19

References

Listerud J, Einstein S, Outwater E, Kressel HY. First principles of fast spin echo. Magn Reson Q. 1992;8:199–244

FSPGR

A GE sequence, abbreviated from Fast SPoiled GRadient echo. A rapid gradient-echo sequence utilizing *spoiling*. The Siemens version of this sequence is called *FLASH*.

FT

Abbreviation for *Fourier Transformation*. Also used on *DICOM* images to denote either Fluoroscopy Trigger or Full echo Train.

Functional MRI

1. When applied to the brain, functional MRI (written as *fMRI*) specifically refers to the techniques for evaluating cortical activation.
2. Also refers generally to any advanced MR method, which permits the examination of function rather than anatomy e.g., perfusion, diffusion, MRS.

Functool

A post-processing package from GE for the analysis of MRI data.

Fusion

Term used to describe the process of merging data from two different imaging modalities in order to display the combined diagnostic information of each technique. Examples include PET-CT and PET-MR to provide functional and anatomical information or MR-CT for soft-tissue detail combined with electron density information for *radiotherapy planning*. Fusion is a aspecific application of image *registration*, requiring similar anatomical landmarks to be present in each image. The two images are usually displayed simultaneously by altering the user defined *transparency* which controls the degree to which each data set is visible.

FUTE

Acronym for Fat suppressed *Ultra-short TE*.

FWHM

Abbreviation for the Full Width at Half Maximum height. This is a common measure of the width of a signal peak. In quality assurance the FWHM of a pixel profile taken along an angled plate is used to measure the slice thickness (see *profile phantom*).

In MRS, the FWHM of the spectral peaks (referred to specifically as *linewidth*) is an indication of *shim* quality. Small values indicate good uniformity and better spectral resolution. Desirable values for FWHM are <7 Hz for single voxel MRS, 10–12 Hz for 2D MRS and <15 Hz for 3D MRSI.

G

G/cm

The unit of magnetic field gradient (*Gauss* per centimeter).
See also *mT/m*.

GABA

Acronym for Gamma-AminoButyric Acid. A brain metabolite with proton MRS peaks at 1.9, 2.3 and 3.0 ppm from the α, δ and γ CH_2 groups (see chemical structure below). The 3.0 ppm peak is usually obscured by creatine but can be seen with *spectral editing*. GABA is an amino acid that acts as an inhibitory neurotransmitter. It may be useful in monitoring the treatment of epilepsy with the drug vigabatin (Fig. 37).

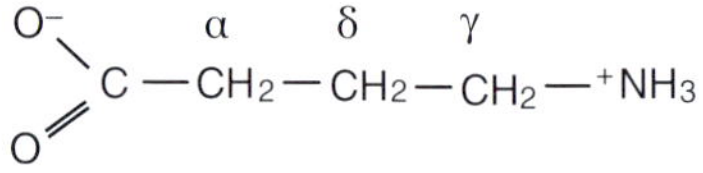

FIGURE 37 The chemical structure of *GABA* illustrating the positions of the α, δ and γ protons

Godobenate dimeglumine

Name of a contrast agent commercially known as *MultiHance*.

Gadobutrol

Name of a contrast agent commercially known as *Gadovist*.

Gadodiamide

Name of a contrast agent commercially known as *Omniscan*.

Gadofosveset trisodium

Name of a contrast agent commercially known as *Vasovist*.

Gadolite

Common name for gadolinium zeolite, an *oral contrast agent*.

Gadolinium

A rare-earth metal with chemical symbol Gd and named after Johan Gadolin. It is strongly paramagnetic and its solutions are widely used as an *exogenous* MR *contrast agent*. It must be chelated to some other molecule (known as a ligand) to reduce its toxicity. This reduces the *relaxivity* of the Gd^{3+} ion, from approximately 10 $mM^{-1}s^{-1}$, to half this value. Of the many agents that currently exist, *Gd-DTPA* has been in the longest clinical use.

Gadomer-17

A *blood pool agent* with a commercial name of Gadomer.

Gadoteridol

Name of the contrast agent known commercially as *ProHance*.

Gadoversetamide

Name of the contrast agent known commercially as *OptiMARK*.

Gadovist

A relatively new contrast agent with the chemical name Gd-DO3A-butriol (Bayer Schering Pharma AG). It is a double osmolar agent and can be used in *contrast-enhanced MRA* to improve the visualization of small vessels.

Gamma

Greek symbol (γ) often used to represent the *gyromagnetic ratio*.

GastroMARK

Another brand name for the contrast agent ferumoxsil (see *Lumirem*).

Gating

Referring to the synchronization of the imaging sequence to some periodicity for example the cardiac cycle or respiratory motion. Cardiac gating is performed with *ECG gating* or *peripheral pulse gating*.

Gating is used to reduce artifacts caused by motion but at the expense of increased imaging time.

See also *respiratory gating*.

Gauss

A small unit of magnetic field strength, where $1\,T = 10,000\,G$. Magnetic field may be measured with a gaussmeter. A hand-held probe may be used having first been calibrated in a zero Gauss screened chamber, to measure a scanner's *fringe field*.

See also *Earth's magnetic field*.

Gaussian

A bell-shaped curve used in statistics to describe a normal (or Gaussian) distribution of data. It is characterized by 65% of the data lying within one standard deviation of the mean value. Gaussian noise refers to a (normal) random distribution of noise.

A Gaussian (shaped) filter is often used in *apodisation,* and is described by the function:

$$G(t) = e^{-t^2/_D}$$

Gd-BOPTA

Chemical name of a contrast agent known commercially as *MultiHance.*

Gd-DTPA

A common MRI contrast agent with the longest safety record of all the agents currently in use. It consists of a *gadolinium* ion chelated to three diethylenetriamine pentaacetic acid (DTPA) producing a linear ionic complex with a –2 charge shown in Fig. 38. This is chemically balanced with two meglumine charges. The resulting agent is called *dimeglumine gadopentetate* and is marketed commercially as *Magnevist.*

Two other contrast agents based on Gd and DTPA are Gd-DTPA-BMA (*Omniscan*) and Gd-DTPA-BMEA (*OptiMARK*).

See also *relaxivity.*

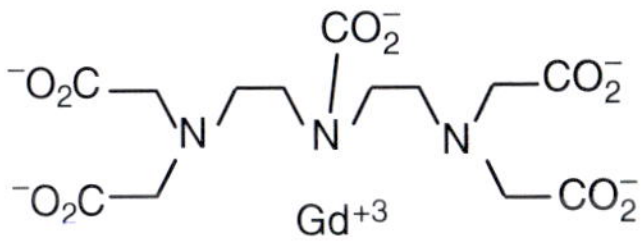

FIGURE 38 The chemical structure of *Gd-DTPA*

References

Nelson KL, Gifford LM, Lauber-Huber C, et al. Clinical safety of dimeglumine gadopentetate. Radiology. 1995;196:439–443

Gd-DOTA

An ionic *gadolinium* based contrast agent. Gadolinium is chelated to tetraaza-cyclododecane-tertraacetic acid (DOTA) to form a cyclic molecule. The resulting agent is called gadoterate, and is marketed as *Dotarem*.

See also *Prohance*.

GE (HealthCare)

One of the leading MRI vendors. Current products include 1.5 T (Signa HDx, MR450 and MR450 *wide bore*) and 3.0 T (Signa HDx & MR750, See Fig. 48) whole body systems, with HD denoting high-density and referring to the number of receiver channels. Open systems (see *open scanner*) include a 0.35 T permanent magnet (Ovation) and an open 0.7 T superconducting system (OpenSpeed).

www.gehealthcare.com

Gel dosimetry

See *MR dosimetry*.

Gel phantoms

One of the *Eurospin test objects* used to investigate relaxation time measurement accuracy and image contrast. It consists of a set of test tubes filled with *agarose gel* doped with varying amounts of *Gd-DTPA* to give a characteristic range of relaxation times (Shown on the right of Fig. 66).

Known values for T_1 and T_2 are determined with MRS and these can be compared with various imaging techniques.

Specific types of gel phantoms are also used in *MR dosimetry*.

See also *quality assurance* and *test object.*

Gelatin

A jelly-like substance derived from animal skin and bones. It can be used as an alternative to *agarose gel* for the construction of phantoms although it has a much lower melting point.

GEM

Abbreviation for Generalized Encoding Matrix. A GE *parallel imaging* sequence, which combines the calibration scan into a single acquisition to reduce scan time. This is a k-space based reconstruction method.

Geometric distortion

A specific measure of distortion related to the change in image shape. A suitable phantom comprising of a grid arrangement of known dimensions may be imaged in order to assess this. Measurements of at least three distances across the phantom are taken and the percentage ratio of the SD to the mean of these measurements is recorded. The acceptable tolerance for routine imaging is ±0.6%.

Distortion is principally caused by changes in B_0 or gradient linearity. The influence of the latter can be reduced by using a high bandwidth (>32 KHz).

Certain sequences are more likely to exhibit distortion (for example *EPI*) (Fig. 39).

See also *linearity.*

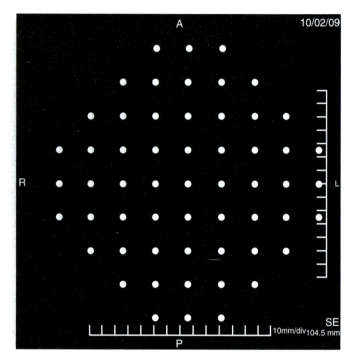

FIGURE 39 An image of a *geometric distortion* phantom comprising of a perspex insert with holes drilled at 25 mm intervals and placed in an aqueous solution. Measurements between the known distances can be used to quantify the distortion of the system

References

Moore CS, Liney GP, Beavis AW. Quality assurance of CT and MR registration for radiotherapy planning of head and neck cancers. Clin Oncol. 2003;15(2):S8

Ghosting

A diffuse or discrete signal artifact that appears throughout the image and is usually caused by patient movement during the scan. Due to the discrepancy in the length of time required for phase and frequency encoding it is predominantly observed in the phase direction. Usually non-periodic motion (coughing etc.) causes a smeared effect while periodic motion (e.g., breathing) appears more discontinuous. It may also be caused by system instability and should be checked as part of *quality assurance* of the scanner. Ghosting is measured in the image background in the phase encoding direction and is expressed as a percentage of the main signal. Acceptable levels are <1% for conventional sequences. Certain sequences exhibit *Nyquist ghosting* (for example *EPI*) which may produce levels of 5% or greater (Fig. 40).

See also *gating*.

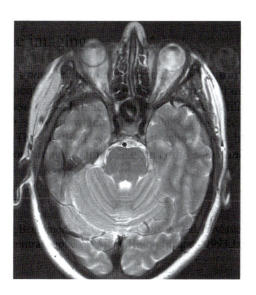

FIGURE 40 *Ghosting* in this image has been caused by movement of the eyeballs during the scan. The artifact is along the phase encoding direction which is right to left. Liney G. MRI in clinical practice. London: Springer; 2006, p. 43

Gibb's artifact

The presence of multiple lines near a high contrast interface which is a consequence of the finite sampling of the analog signal. It is commonly seen in the C-spine. It is usually associated with the *phase encoding* direction as this is the matrix which is often reduced to limit *acquisition time*. It is also referred to as *truncation artifact* or ringing (Fig. 41).

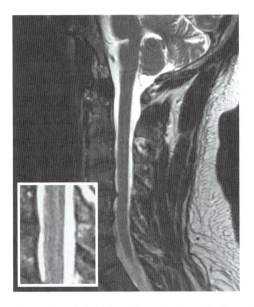

FIGURE 41 Example of *Gibb's artifact* in the spinal cord (shown magnified in *inset*). Liney G. MRI in clinical practice. London: Springer; 2006, p. 42

Gibb's overshoot

The oscillations at the edge of a square waveform when only a finite number of harmonics are used in its representation. It is the cause of *Gibbs artifact* in MR images.

See also *Fourier transformation*.

GKM

Abbreviation for General Kinetic Model. Software used to standardize the *pharmacokinetic modeling* of dynamic contrast enhanced data.

Glx

Notation used in proton spectra to indicate the combined peaks of glutamate (Glu) and glutamine (Gln), which are not readily resolved at field strengths of less than 4.0 T. Peaks occur at 2.0–2.4 ppm and 3.6–3.8 ppm. Levels in the brain have been observed to increase in liver failure.

The chemical structure of glutamate is shown in Fig. 42. In Glutamine the O^- ion at the right hand end is replaced with NH_2.

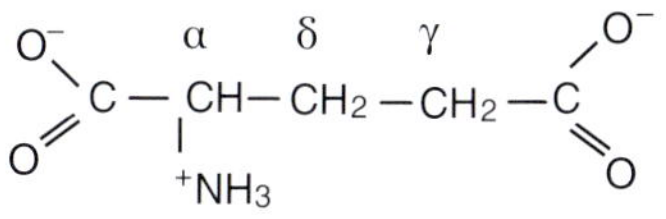

FIGURE 42 The chemical structure of *glutamate*

Glutamate, glutamine

Brain metabolites seen in proton MRS.
See also Glx.

Goggles

Fiber-optic based video equipment used to provide a visual stimulus (or instructions) in functional MRI (*fMRI*) experiments. These provide a potentially more reliable alternative to the use of a projection screen which is viewed via the mirror in the RF head coil.

Golay coils

Design of a *gradient coil* consisting of a set of four coils lying along the scanner bore to produce the transverse gradients (G_x and G_y). This corresponds to a linear field change in a direction perpendicular to the B_0. A diagram of a Golay coil is shown in Fig. 43.

See also *Maxwell pair*.

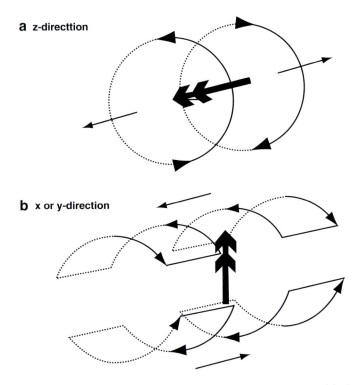

a z-directtion

b x or y-direction

FIGURE 43 Two types of *gradient coil* used in the scanner. (**a**) A Maxwell pair is used to vary the field in the z-direction. (**b**) Two sets of Golay coils, one rotated at 90° from the other, are used to produce the x or y gradients. The directions of the current (*arrow*), magnetic field (*thin arrow*), and gradient (*double arrow*) is shown in each case

Gradient

A linear change in magnetic field produced by a *gradient coil*. The application of a gradient results in a change of both phase and frequency and this was first proposed by Lauterbur as a method of encoding an image. Gradient specifications are given in terms of peak amplitude and *rise time*, or as a combined *slew rate*. Typical gradient amplitudes are 10–50 mT m^{-1}.

References

Lauterbur PC. Image formation by induced local interactions: examples employing nuclear magnetic resonance. Nature. 1973;242:190–191

Gradient area

The product of amplitude and duration of an imaging gradient. It is represented schematically by the rectangular areas drawn in a *pulse sequence diagram*.

Gradient coil

Part of the MRI scanner that produces a magnetic field *gradient* in a particular direction. There are three separate gradient coils in the scanner (termed a *Maxwell pair* and *Golay coils*). These can produce a gradient in each orthogonal direction or are used in combination to produce *oblique* gradient directions. They must be shielded to prevent *eddy currents*. Any non-linearities in the gradients will result in *geometric distortion* (Fig. 43).

Gradient echo

Also known as gradient recalled echo. A type of MR signal created by the application of a gradient reversal. Unlike a *spin-echo*,

it is characterized by the absence of a 180° *refocusing pulse* leading to shorter repetition times and faster sequences. This also
makes the signal inherently T_2* *weighted* and prone to susceptibility artifacts.

For a spoiled gradient echo sequence the signal is given
by:

$$S \propto \frac{\sin \alpha \left(1 - \exp\left(-TR/T_1\right)\right)\exp\left(TE/T_2^*\right)}{1 - \cos \alpha \exp(-TR/T_1)}$$

where α is the flip angle (Fig. 44).

See also *partial flip* and *spoiling*.

Gradient moment nulling

Reduction of flow effects by using gradients to ensure signal
is re-phased appropriately. Also known as Motion Artifact
Suppression Technique (*MAST*), or flow compensation (FC)
and implemented by Fonar as STILL.

See also *even echo rephasing* and *flow compensation*.

Graphic prescription

Referring to the use of a visual display of a previously
acquired image or images to assist in the manual positioning
of slices or voxel locations used in subsequent scans.

GRAPPA

Siemens k-space based implementation of *parallel imaging*. It
is an acronym for GeneRalized Autocalibrating Partially
Parallel Acquisition.

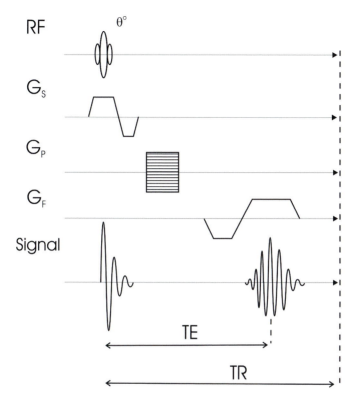

FIGURE 44 Pulse sequence diagram for the *gradient echo* sequence. G_S, G_P and G_F represent the gradients for the slice selection, phase encoding and frequency encoding respectively. The hatched lines of G_P indicate that this amplitude is varied incrementally for each TR. In contrast to a spin-echo sequence (shown in Fig. 88) there is no 180° pulse and the excitation pulse is shown as $\theta°$ to indicate a variable flip angle. Liney G. MRI in clinical practice. London: Springer; 2006, p. 18

References

Griswold MA, Jakob PM, Heidemann RM, et al. A generalised autocalibrating partially parallel acquisitions (GRAPPA). Magn Reson Med. 2002;47:1202–1210

GRASE

Acronym for GRAdient and Spin Echo. A hybrid sequence that acquires alternate gradient and spin-echoes. The final signal has an intermediate contrast effect. The sequence has been used as an alternative to *EPI*.

GRASS

Acronym for Gradient Recalled Acquisition in Steady State. A GE *steady state* sequence.

GRACE

Acronym from GeneRalized breAst speCtroscopy Exam. A Siemens product for quantitative *choline* spectroscopy in the breast. The technique uses either the signal from water as an internal concentration reference or from an external sample which is housed in the breast coil itself.

Grayscale

The normal representation of image data. A color map is assigned to the pixel values with the minimum value set to black and the maximum value set to white. All other values are assigned intermediate shades of gray. For an *inverse image* the opposite scale is used. Alternatively a user-defined color scale may be used (e.g., "hot iron"-a yellow/orange scale is often used in fMRI to display activated pixels). Often *parameter maps* are shown in color and overlaid onto the original grayscale images.

Gyromagnetic ratio

The property of a nucleus that determines its resonant frequency and related to its mass and charge. It is the constant in the *Larmor equation* (denoted as γ), and is alternatively called the magnetogyric ratio. Hydrogen has a value of 42.58 MHz T^{-1}.

$G_z (G_x, G_y)$

Notation used to indicate a gradient in the z- (or x,y) direction. A *Maxwell pair* is used to produce G_z and two sets of *Golay coils* are used for G_x and G_y. These are shown in Fig. 43. The gradients are turned on in a specific order depending on how they are used (e.g., see Fig. 88).

H

h

Letter used to denote Planck's constant (equal to 6.626×10^{-34} J s). A physical constant that relates the energy and frequency of an electromagnetic wave. It is often written as $\hbar$ (pronounced "h-bar") which is Planck's constant divided by 2π, also known as Dirac's constant. This is used to express *angular frequency* in *radians* per second. The energy difference between the *spin-up* and spin-down state is given by:

$$\Delta E = \hbar \omega_o$$

where ω_0 is the *larmor frequency*.
 See also *Boltzmann distribution*.

Hemodynamic lag

The delay between actual neuronal activation and the time taken for increased oxygen demand to be observed with *BOLD* fMRI. The difference is of the order of several seconds.
 See also *haemodynamic response function*.

Hemodynamic response function

A function which is convolved with the *fMRI* stimulus pattern to take into account the expected haemodynamic delay. This produces a more physiologically realistic reference waveform that can be used to compare with the signal response.

Hahn echo

A particular spin-echo sequence where the excitation and refocusing flip angles differ from the optimum 90° and 180° used normally. The reduced signal is related to the two flip angles α_1 and α_2 by:

$$\sin \alpha_1 \sin^2 (\alpha_2 / 2)$$

References

Hahn EL. Spin echoes. Phys Rev. 1950;80:589–594

Half echo

Alternative name for *partial echo*.

Half scan

Alternative name for *partial Fourier*.

Halo artifact

A strange appearance where the signal at the center of the image appears washed out and the background signal is bright. It occurs whenever the receiver gain is incorrectly set (see *over-ranging*) and the measured signal becomes truncated (Fig. 45).

Hanning filter

A type of low pass spatial domain filter. It is a symmetrical function characterized by high values at the center and a cosine-shaped roll-off, given by:

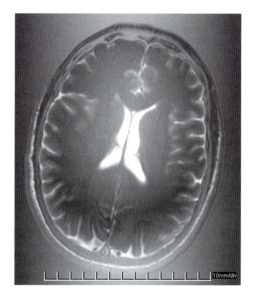

<small>FIGURE 45</small> A brain image demonstrating a *halo artifact* due to the RF amplifier over-ranging. Liney G. MRI in clinical practice. London: Springer; 2006, p. 49

$$H(x) = 0.5 + 0.5(\cos 2\pi x / I)$$

where I is the width of the Hanning window (smaller values cause a sharper roll-off).

See also *low-pass filtering* and *high-pass filtering*.

HARP

Abbreviation for HARmonic Phase. An automated method of analyzing tagged images in cardiac MRI using image filtering in order to speed up the analysis of myocardial motion.

See also *spin tagging*.

HASTE

Acronym for HAlf-Fourier Single-shot Turbo spin Echo. A sequence based on the FSE technique in which only half of k-space is acquired thereby improving imaging speed. It is often used in abdominal imaging to reduce motion artifacts.

See also *partial k-space*.

Head coil

The RF *transceiver* coil used in the imaging of head and brain anatomy. It is usually a *birdcage* design and comprises some sort of adjustable mirror so the patient can see outside of the magnet bore. Some types have attachable anterior neck elements to increase coverage inferiorly (more commonly known as head-and-neck coils). In certain situations where space is limited (e.g., in *radiotherapy planning*) dedicated flexible coils may be used instead (Fig. 46).

See also *RF coil*.

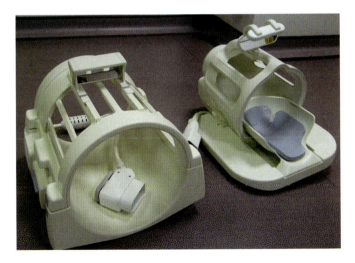

FIGURE 46 Photograph of (*left*) a linear RF *head coil* and (*right*) a smaller 8-channel version from GE Healthcare

Head first entry

Method of positioning the patient in the scanner for imaging the head and upper torso.

See also *feet first entry*.

Header

The information part of an image file, which is gives details concerning patient name, date and scanning sequence etc rather than the pixel intensity values. The header will be either of fixed length or contain the starting position (in number of bytes) of the subsequent image data.

See also *DICOM*.

Heat exchanger

A device built for the efficient heat transfer from one medium to another. A heat exchanger is used to control the supply of water to the *cold head* compressor and also the water which is used to cool the gradients.

Helium

Inert gas and second lightest element with an extremely low boiling point ($-269°C$). It is used in liquid form as the *cryogen* for a superconducting scanner.

Helium has an MR visible isotope (^{3}He) with a very low natural abundance, meaning it is mostly sourced as a nuclear decay product. It is inherently sensitive, but its low spin density means its signal is too weak to be used without first being hyperpolarised (see *hyperpolarized gas imaging*).

MR properties of ^{3}He:

Spin quantum number $= 1/2$
Sensitivity $= 0.44$

Natural abundance = 0.000137%
Gyromagnetic ratio = 32.43 MHz T^{-1}.

Helmholtz pair

An arrangement of two magnetic coils with the separation distance equal to their radius, producing a very uniform field.
  See also *solenoid*.

Hepatobiliary agents

Type of MRI contrast agents that are taken up by hepatocytes in the normal liver.
  See also *liver-specific contrast agents.*

Hermitian symmetry

Referring to the diagonal (or *conjugate*) symmetry that occurs in k-space.

Herringbone artifact

A characteristic criss-cross pattern appearance in the image due to a data reconstruction error. The artifact is present in every pixel due to the nature of *k-space*. It is also sometimes referred to as a corduroy artifact (Fig. 47).

Hertz

The unit of frequency, where 1 Hz is equal to 1 cycle per second (s^{-1}). Note that *angular frequency* is given in *radians* per second (rad s^{-1}).

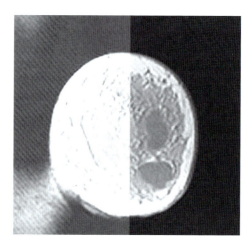

FIGURE 47 Example breast image demonstrating a *herringbone arti-fact*. Half of the image has been windowed differently to show that the effect propagates throughout the whole image. Liney G. MRI in clinical practice. London: Springer; 2006, p. 51

Heteronuclear correlation spectroscopy

A form of 2D spectroscopy involving two different nuclear spins, usually proton and one other e.g., carbon.
  See also *COSY*.

HIFUS

Acronym for High Intensity Focused UltraSound. A technique used to thermally ablate tumors under MR guidance. It is also used to shrink intrauterine fibroids.
  See also *MR thermometry*.

High field

Loosely defined as a magnetic field strength of 3.0 T and above. Currently clinical scanners are limited to 3.0 T, although research scanners operate at fields of up to 11.0 T. An *open scanner* may be termed "high field" at much lower strengths of around 1.0 T (Fig. 48).

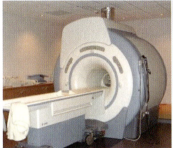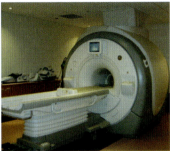

FIGURE 48 Two different *high field* systems (*left*). A 3.0 T HDx system and (*right*) a newer 3.0 T MR750, both from GE Healthcare. The quench pipe can be seen separately to the cold head on the older system

High order phase

Referring to the high amplitude phase encoding steps, which correspond to the data at the edges of *k-space* and determine the spatial detail in the image.

High pass filtering

The removal of low frequency components from MR data. In MRS, it may be used to remove *residual water* from a spectrum, preserving the higher frequency metabolite peaks. The filter consists of the value 1 above a certain frequency threshold and zero elsewhere.

See also *low pass filtering*.

High velocity signal loss

Phenomenon of flowing blood in a spin-echo sequence, which can be used as an *MRA* technique. Blood appears dark (*black-blood*) as it moves out of the imaging slice between the 90° and 180° RF pulses, due to the signal not being refocused.

The velocity, v, needed to exit the slice and produce the maximum signal loss, is given by:

$$v > d / (TE/2)$$

where d is slice thickness.

Higher order shimming

See *active shimming*.

Hitachi (Medical Systems)

MRI vendor currently offering a 1.5 T whole-body scanner (called Echelon), a 0.3 T permanent scanner (AIRIS), and an open 1.2 T vertical field superconducting system (Oasis).

www.hitachimed.com

HOAST

Acronym for High Order Active Shimming Technology used by Hitachi.

See also *shim* and *active shimming*.

Homogeneity

The uniformity of the magnetic field over the imaging volume. This can refer to either the main magnetic field (see B_0

inhomogeneity) or the RF field, where variations lead to incorrect flip angles (see B_1 *inhomogeneity*).

Horizontal bore

The conventional type of MRI system where the magnetic field runs parallel to the patient in the head-to-foot direction.
    See also *vertical bore*.

HRF

Abbreviation for *Haemodynamic Response Function*.

Hybrid systems

Referring to MRI scanners that are combined with a second modality. Examples include *PET*-MRI and *Linac*-MRI. Systems also exist where the patient tables are extended with a C-arm X-ray unit mounted at the opposite end.

Hydrogen

The lightest element with an atomic number equal to 1, and exists in normal conditions as a gaseous molecule (dihydrogen). Its most common isotope ^{1}H (protium) consists of a single *proton* and is the mostly exploited of all the MR visible nuclei due to its high abundance and sensitivity.
    MR properties of ^{1}H:

Spin quantum number = 1/2
Sensitivity = 1.0000
Natural abundance = 99.98%
Gyromagnetic ratio = 42.57 MHz T^{-1}

See also *deuterium*.

Hyperechoes

A symmetrical distribution of equally spaced reduced *flip angle* pulses either side of a 180° pulse (i.e., α_1 and $-\alpha_1$). The contribution of *stimulated echo* components in the hyperecho formation provides increased signal intensity over that obtained from a conventional sequence. The use of the low flip angles makes the sequence less *SAR* intensive compared to conventional FSE sequences and is useful at high field.

References

Hennig J, Scheffler K. Hyperechoes. Magn Reson Med. 2001;46:6–12

Hyperintense

Description of signal intensity, which is brighter than surrounding tissue (see Fig. 94).

See also *hypointense* and *isointense*.

Hyperpolarization

The process of increasing the signal from a low sensitivity MR visible nuclei by several orders of magnitude (for example ^{13}C, ^{15}N, ^{3}He) with yields typically around 20–40%. Various methods exist including *dynamic nuclear polarization* and *parahydrogen-induced polarization*.

See also *hyperpolarised gas imaging*.

Hyperpolarized gas imaging

The use of a laser-polarized MR visible gas (e.g., *xenon*, *helium*) in lung *ventilation imaging*. The normally weak signal is improved by hyperpolarisation using *optical pumping* techniques, which can increase the signal by a factor of 100,000. This increase is sufficient for the gas itself to be imaged.

An additional advantage of xenon is that it dissolves in the blood and can be used in a combined ventilation/perfusion exam.

References

Fain SB, Korosec FR, Holmes JH, O'Halloran R, Sorkness RL, Grist TM. Functional lung imaging using hyperpolarized gas MRI. J Magn Reson Imaging. 2007;25:910–923

Hypointense

Description of signal intensity, which is darker than surrounding tissue (see Fig. 92).

See also *hyperintense* and *isointense*.

Hypoxia

The reduction of oxygen supply to a tissue. On a cellular level, the oxygen deficiency of hypoxic tumors increases their resistance to radiotherapy and chemotherapy and makes them more likely to metastasise. The gold standard measurement is via oxygen partial pressure using an Eppendorf electrode, which involves inserting a needle into the tumor. MRI may also be used to measure hypoxia and techniques include spectroscopy (via the detection of *lactate*), contrast enhancement (perfusion) and R_2^* mapping.

I

I

Letter used to denote the spin *quantum number*.

IAM

Abbreviation for Internal Auditory Meatus. The small canal through the temporal lobe containing facial and auditory nerves, which can imaged with a high-resolution T_2-weighted sequence.

IAPS

Acronym for International Affective Picture System. A database of photographs (University of Florida) that standardize a range of emotions for use in *fMRI* experiments.

ICD

Abbreviation for Implantable Cardioverter Defibrillator. A medical device that is designed to detect and treat ventricular fibrillation. These devices should be treated in the same way as *pacemakers*.

IDEAL

Acronym for Iterative Decomposition of water and fat with Echo Asymmetry and Least squares estimation. A GE sequence based on a three-point *DIXON* technique. The sequence can be used to produce an *in-phase image*, *out-of-phase image*, *water-only image* and *fat-only image*. It also utilizes a B_0 correction map making it more robust to inhomogeneity.

See also *chemical shift ("of the second kind")* and *OOPS*.

References

Reeder SB, Pineda AR, Wen ZF, et al. Iterative decomposition of water and fat with echo asymmetry and least squares estimation (IDEAL): application with fast spin-echo imaging. Magn Reson Med. 2005;54:636–644

Image registration

See *registration*.

Imaginary

1. The non-real part of a complex number.
2. Also the name given to one of the two signal components from a *quadrature* coil and usually denoted as Q (Quadrature).

    See also *real*.

Imaging, 2D

The standard method of image acquisition which utilizes *slice selection* to acquire multiple 2D planar images. Typically, the in-plane *spatial resolution* is 1 mm or better. The through-plane (or slice) resolution is usually limited to around 3–5 mm. Images may still be reformatted and displayed in 3D although best results are obtained with thin *contiguous* slices or true 3D acquisitions.

See also *phase encoding* and *frequency encoding*.

Imaging, 3D

Definition of an image acquisition where a volume or *slab* is acquired and this is subdivided into thin sections using *phase encoding* in the "slice" direction. This has the advantage over multiple 2D imaging in terms of improved through-plane resolution, which is usually of the order of 1–2 mm. This provides more *isotropic* images which can be reformatted or displayed in 3D with good quality.

In addition signal-to-noise ratio (see *SNR*) improves by a factor of $\sqrt{N}$ where N is the number of phase encoding steps in the slice direction. The penalty is increased scan time, which increases linearly with N.

Phase wrap in 3D imaging has to be also considered in the slice direction (see *moire fringes*). On some systems, additional images are acquired in the slice direction and these are discarded to prevent signal wrap affecting the prescribed volume.

Impedance matching

Ensuring that the electrical impedance (resistance, inductance and capacitance) of the coil is commensurate with ancillary electronic components. This ensures that RF energy is efficiently transferred between the system and the coil.

See also *cable-loss*.

Implants

See *MR compatible*, *deflection angle test* and *silicon*.

iMRI

Abbreviation for Interventional MRI (note the lower-case i by convention). Referring to any MR examination where hardware (e.g., RF coils or the magnet bore) is specifically designed to permit some interventional procedure to be performed on the patient under MR guidance.

See also *interventional device*, *MR guided* and *open scanner*.

Infarct penumbra

A circumferential region in the area of reduced diffusion seen in stroke, which may still be viable and demonstrates normal perfusion characteristics in MRI.

See also *perfusion imaging*.

Inferior

The conventional direction of the patient's feet and the opposite direction to *superior*. It is towards the bottom of a *sagittal* and *coronal* image (see Figs. 18 and 82.)

In-flow enhancement

Also known as flow-related enhancement. The phenomenon of flowing blood entering the slice in gradient echo imaging making it appear bright. Repeated RF pulses *saturate* stationary spins whereas fresh spins entering the slice for the first time are fully magnetized and appear bright. The first slice usually demonstrates the greatest enhancement (leading to the alternative name of entry-slice phenomenon). The effect is reduced as slice thickness is increased, but this can be overcome by using a variable *flip angle* across the imaging slice (see *TONE*).

In order to produce a maximum enhancement these spins need continually replacing in-between successive RF pulses. This means a velocity equal to d/TR where d is the slice thickness.

Infusion pump

A device for the automatic delivery of *contrast agents* ensuring a reproducible dose. The volume and rate of delivery can be set, and the device is operated from inside the control room.

InHance

A non-contrast enhanced MRA sequence from GE. Other similar sequences include TRANCE (Philips), NATIVE (Siemens), VASC (Hitachi) and FBI/CIA (Toshiba).

Inorganic phosphate

A spectral peak seen at 5.0 ppm in *phosphorus* MRS. The change in its chemical shift can also be used to calculate pH from the Henderson-Hasselbach equation (see Fig. 70).

In-phase image

An image acquired at a specific echo time so that the water and fat signal are in phase. An example of an in-phase image is shown in Fig. 10.

   See also *chemical shift* (*"of the second kind"*) and *fat-water in-phase*.

Integrated body coil

See *body coil*.

Intensity correction

See *coil uniformity correction*.

Interleaved

The acquisition of alternative or non-*sequential* slices i.e., "odd" numbered slices are followed by "even" numbered slices. This is performed as a method of eliminating *cross excitation*.

Interpolation

Estimation of an intermediate data point from a series of data points. Image interpolation refers to the process of improving spatial resolution by increasing the image matrix and filling in the missing points from some manipulation of the intensity values in adjacent rows and columns. Common interpolation methods include nearest neighbor, linear or cubic spline. The opposite process is called decimation.

Interventional device

MR compatible device, which permits an MR guided interventional procedure to be performed (e.g., a biopsy). The device should consist of fiducial markers, which are visible on MRI and subsequently enable the localisation of anatomy with respect to an external co-ordinate system (Fig. 49).

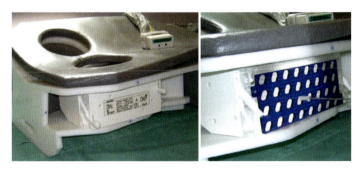

FIGURE 49 An example of an *interventional device* used in conjunction with an open breast coil (MACHNET, The Netherlands) to enable MR guided biopsy or wire localisation

References

Liney GP, Tozer DJ, van Hulten HB, Beerens EG, et al. Bilateral open breast coil and compatible intervention device. J Magn Reson Imaging. 2000;12:984–990

Inverse lateralization

Referring to the activation observed in motor and sensory fMRI experiments, which appears in the opposite hemisphere to the side of the patient being tested (i.e., left motor cortex corresponds to right hand movement).

Inversion pulse

An *excitation pulse* using a 180° flip angle in order to invert the spins so that they are aligned along the negative *z-direction*.

Inversion recovery

Abbreviated to IR. The use of an *inversion pulse* so that T_1 recovery of the magnetization begins along the negative z direction.

The technique is often used as a method of fat or water suppression e.g., *STIR, FLAIR*.

Inversion recovery sequences may also be used to measure T_1 by varying the inversion time (see *TI*). Signal is given by:

$$S \propto \left[1 - 2\exp(-TI/T_1) + \exp(-TR/T_1)\right]\exp(-TE/T_2)$$

Which can be simplified when $TR \gg T_1$ to:

$$S \propto \left[1 - 2\exp(-TI/T_1)\right]$$

Several repeat measurements need be made covering a suitable range of inversion times for the expected T_1 value making it a lengthy process.

Sometimes inversion recovery sequences are prefixed with the words "real" or "true" to indicate that the non-magnitude signal is reconstructed which extends the contrast range.

See also *short tau inversion recovery*, *null-point* and *bounce-point artifact*.

Inversion time

See *TI* and *inversion recovery*.

Inverse image

Displaying the image with an inverted *grayscale* i.e., black for the maximum value, and white for the minimum value. This is useful when comparing MR Angiography results with conventional digital subtraction angiography (see *DSA*).

IPA

Acronym for Integrated Panoramic Arrays. A Siemens term referring to the connectability of various RF coils and now more commonly known as Total Imaging Matrix (see *TIM*).

iPAT

Acronym for Integrated Parallel Acquisition Technique. The name for Siemens' package of *parallel imaging* sequences. This includes an image based reconstruction method (mSENSE) and a k-space method (*GRAPPA*).

See also *SENSE*.

IR

Abbreviation for *Inversion recovery*, and used as a prefix in sequences to indicate that these are inversion *prepared* i.e., they begin with the magnetization along the negative z-direction.

IRM

Abbreviation for Inversion Recovery Magnitude. This is used to indicate that the magnitude component of the inverted signal is being utilized.

Ischemia

Term relating to insufficient blood supply to a particular organ. Ischemia leads to *hypoxia*, which refers specifically to oxygen deficiency. Ischemia in the brain can lead to *stroke* which may be readily identified on diffusion weighted sequences (see *DWI*).

ISIS

Acronym for Image Selected In vivo Spectroscopy. A method of spectroscopy localisation, which involves combinations of non-selective and selective inversion pulses. These are then algebraically combined to obtain the desired signal.

Isocenter

The central point inside the scanner bore, which, by definition is the most homogenous part of the magnetic field. The patient is landmarked prior to scanning and moved so that point is moved to the isocenter. Each subsequent image prescription will re-position the patient according to the change in relation to the isocenter.

See also *DSV*.

Isochromat

Referring to spins that have the same precessional frequency (Literally meaning same color).

Isointense

Description of signal intensity which appears the same as surrounding tissue.

See also *hypointense* and *hyperintense*.

Isotope

Chemical element of the same species having the same number of protons (atomic number) but a different mass number i.e., varies in the number of neutrons.

Isotropic

Usually referring to spatial resolution, which is equivalent in all three orthogonal directions. This is crucial for good quality reformatting (see *reformat*) and 3D reconstructions.

Also used to describe diffusion, which has the same magnitude in each direction (see *anisotropy*).

J

J-coupling

The phenomenon of spin-spin interaction mediated by cova-
lent bonds (usually the nearest), which leads to splitting of
spectral peaks. Also known as indirect or scalar coupling. The
magnitude of the effect is given by the coupling constant, J,
and molecules exhibiting this are subdivided into *AX systems*
or *AB* systems.

See also *TE averaging* and *COSY.*

J-modulation

See *echo modulation*.

JET

Name given to Toshiba's *radial k-space* technique for motion
compensation.

Joule

The unit of energy. It is defined as the energy exerted by a
force of 1 N in order to move an object 1 m or 1 W of power
for 1 s.

K

Kaplan–Meier plot

A step-wise plot demonstrating patient survival following a given intervention or treatment. The y-axis shows the proportion of surviving patients and the x-axis gives the survival time.

References

Everitt BS. Medical statistics from A to Z. Cambridge: Cambridge University Press; 2003. ISBN: 0521532043

Key-hole imaging

A *partial k-space* technique where only the central portion of k-space is acquired to speed up imaging time and improve the *temporal resolution*. Image detail is subsequently filled in from a separate scan in which the whole of k-space has been recorded. The method works well when only bulk signal changes from image to image e.g., in *contrast enhanced MRA*.

References

Van Vaals JJ, Brummer ME, Dixon WT. Dixon et al. Keyhole method for imaging of contrast uptake. J Magn Reson Imaging. 1993;3:671–675

Kinematic imaging

Referring to any MRI technique and associated hardware that enables physiological motion to be studied. This may

176 MRI from A to Z

simply involve static imaging in a number of physiologically relevant positions (*positional MRI*) or more accurately refer to real-time imaging as motion takes place.

k-Space

An array of numbers whose 2D *Fourier transformation* produces the MR image. Each element in k-space contains information about every image pixel. The faster k-space can be filled, the quicker the image acquisition. Many techniques are available which speed up imaging by only partially filling k-space, however image quality is degraded. The order in which k-space is filled may be used advantageously and relates to the timing of the *low order phase* or *high order phase* encoding steps.

K refers to the wave-number or wave cycles per unit distance. It is the spatial analog to frequency and is related to the imaging gradients by:

$$k = \gamma Gt$$

where γ is the *gyromagnetic ratio*, G is the amplitude of the encoding gradient and t is the duration of this gradient (the product Gt is the *gradient area*).

The maximum value of k (k_{max}) is the reciprocal of pixel size, and the k-space sampling size (Δk) is the reciprocal of the field-of-view (Fig. 50).

See also *partial k-space*, *k-space trajectory*, *radial k-space* and *conjugate symmetry*.

References

Mezrich R. Perspective on k-space (tutorial). Radiology. 1995;195:297–315

k-Space ordering

The order in which k-space is filled i.e., whether the high or low phase encoding steps are acquired first.

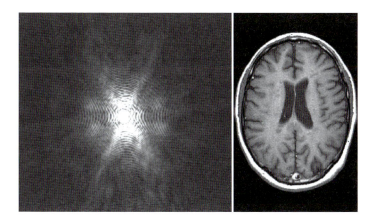

FIGURE 50 *k-Space* data on the left which is Fourier transformed into the image shown on the right. Liney G. MRI in clinical practice. London: Springer; 2006, p. 15

See also *sequential k-space filling* and *centric k-space filling.*

k-Space path

See *k-space trajectory.*

k-Space shutter

A *partial k-space* technique in which the outer lines of k-space are not acquired in order to speed up imaging time. Equivalent to *key-hole imaging.*

k-Space trajectory

Referring to the direction in which k-space is traversed (i.e., how the gradient encoding is performed). The more efficiently this is done, the faster the image can be recorded. The simplest method acquires k-space in a sequential line-by-line fashion (sometimes referred to as *cartesian*), although the ordering may be changed (e.g., *centric k-space*). More complicated approaches include spiral trajectories and radial trajectories are now commonly used to reduce motion artifacts (see *radial k-space*).

k-t BLAST

Acronym for k-space and time-space Broad use Linear Acquisition Speed-up Technique. Exploits the *k-space* and temporal correlations of *dynamic* data ascertained from low-resolution "training" images (for example in cardiac imaging). These are then used in subsequent imaging to speed up acquisition time. A *SENSE* version of this sequence is also available.

References

Tsao J, Boesiger P, Pruessmann KP. k-t BLAST and k-t SENSE: Dynamic MRI with high frame rate exploiting spatiotemporal correlations. Magn Reson Med. 2003;50:1031–1042

K^{TRANS}

Notation used for the Transfer constant. This is a parameter determined from *pharmacokinetic modeling* which describes the exchange of contrast agent between the blood plasma and the extracellular space. Other parameters include V_e, the volume of extracellular space, and K_{ep} or the rate constant, defined as K^{TRANS}/V_e. When the contrast delivery to the tissue is sufficient, the transfer constant is equal to the capillary permeability surface area product (see Fig. 67).

References

Tofts PS, Brix G, et al. Estimating kinetic parameters from dynamic contrast-enhanced T_1-weighted MRI of a diffusible tracer: standardized quantities and symbols. J Magn Reson Imaging. 1999;10:223–232

L

Laboratory frame

A stationary frame of reference where spins precess at the larmor frequency with respect to the observer's point of view. A much simpler *rotating frame* of reference is usually adopted in text books and diagrams to describe the effects of RF pulses.

Lactate

A metabolite in proton MRS, which is related to the end product of anaerobic metabolism and is not usually seen but it may become visible in *hypoxia*. It appears as a doublet and is further characterized by having an inverted peak at an echo time of 135 ms. It has a chemical shift of 1.33 ppm and may be obscured by the main *lipid* signal (Fig. 51).

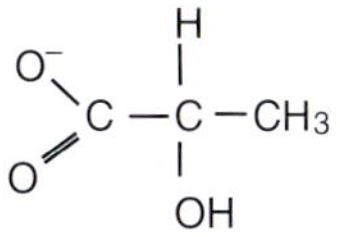

FIGURE 51 The chemical structure of *lactate*

Large field-of-view filter

An image filter used to correct for the *geometric distortion* at the edge of the field-of-view due to inherent B_0 *inhomogeneity*.
    See also *DSV*.

Larmor equation

See *larmor frequency*.

Larmor frequency

The precessional or resonant frequency (ω_0) of a nuclear *spin* when it is placed in an external magnetic field. It is related to the magnetic field (B_0) by the Larmor equation:

$$\omega_0 = \gamma B_0$$

where γ is the *gyromagnetic ratio*. Here, frequency is in *radians* per second. Conventionally written (although strictly incorrect) without a negative sign.

The resonant frequency for protons is 63.8 and 127.7 MHz at 1.5 and 3.0 T respectively.

See also *precession*.

Landmark

Referring to the alignment of the patient with the *isocenter* of the scanner.

Laser

The alignment light projected from the bore entrance of the scanner used to *landmark* the patient prior to scanning.

In some sites where MRI is used for *radiotherapy planning*, an external laser system may also be present. This consists of a goal-post frame attached to the scan room floor and is able project a moveable landmark in each plane to correspond to similar CT landmarks.

Laser ablation

The use of MR-guided laser treatment to destroy tumor tissue. It has been used to good effect in the liver. Also referred to as Laser-Induced Thermotherapy (LITT).

See also *MR thermometry*.

LAVA

Acronym for Liver Acquisition with Volume Acceleration. A 3D gradient-echo sequence from GE. Variants to this include LAVA-XV with accelerated (*ASSET*) imaging and LAVA-Flex with 2-point *DIXON* imaging. Other equivalent sequences include VIBE (from Siemens) and THRIVE (from Philips).

Leksell-frame

A *stereotactic* device attached to the patient's skull for pre-surgical brain MRI. Some RF head coils are specifically designed to accommodate this device together with associated software to correct for any *geometric distortion* that is introduced in the image.

Lenz's law

Law of physics which states that an induced current acts in such a way so that the magnetic field produced opposes the change that caused it. It is responsible for the negative sign in the equation describing *Faraday's law*.

Level

Referring to the intensity or window level of the image display. The center of the *grayscale* range is set to this value.
  See also *windowing*.

LC model

An MRS processing algorithm used to estimate metabolic concentrations (abbreviation of linear combination model). A basis set of spectra created from solutions of known concentrations are combined in order to best fit the acquired data.

References

Provencher S. Estimation of metabolite concentrations from localized in vivo proton NMR spectra. Magn Reson Med. 1993;30:62

Liquid helium

See *helium*.

Linac

Acronym for LINear ACcelerator. A machine that produces
high energy (megavoltage) X-rays and electrons for use in external beam *radiotherapy*. Novel hybrid systems whereby a Linac
and MRI scanner are combined are currently being prototyped.

Line broadening

See *apodisation*.

Linearity

A measure of the change in the image dimensions due to *distortion*. It can be quantified as the absolute difference between
the mean of (at least) three measurements taken in images of
a suitable phantom from the known dimension. Acceptable
tolerance is typically ±1 mm for a distance of 120 mm.
    See also *quality assurance*.

Linear regression

A statistical method used to investigate the relationship
between two groups of variables. More specifically it is used
to predict one variable from the other.

Linearly polarized

The simplest form of RF coil (i.e., a coil that does not operate in *quadrature*). Often abbreviated to LP.

Linewidth

A measure of the spectral peak width, giving an indication of *shim* quality (see *FWHM*). The linewidth is inversely proportional to T_2^*. Narrow linewidths enable closely spaced peaks to be discriminated. The term also specifies the width of the spectral filter used in *apodisation*.

Linguine sign

Term used to describe the coiled low signal intensity appearance resembling a piece of linguine pasta that is seen in MRI of ruptured breast implants.

Lipid

A number of peaks from fatty tissue observed in proton MRS. These are comprised of methylene (CH_2) protons at 1.3 ppm and terminal methyl (CH_3) protons at 0.9 ppm. There are also peaks at 2.06 and 5.35 ppm (from unsaturated lipids). The dominant peak at 1.3 ppm may need suppressing in certain regions (e.g., breast) in order to observe other metabolites (Fig. 52).

References

Jagannathan NR, Singh M, Govindaraju V, et al. Volume localized in vivo proton MR spectroscopy of breast carcinoma: variation of water-fat ratio in patients receiving chemotherapy. NMR Biomed. 1998;11:414–422

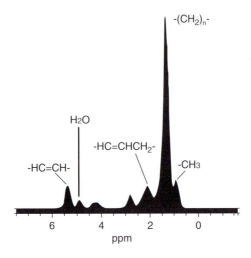

FIGURE 52 Water suppressed MR spectrum of soya oil shows the four *lipid* peaks that may be observed in vivo. The residual water peak is also shown. The remaining fat peaks (not labeled) are not usually seen in vivo

Liposomes

Tiny bubbles composed of phospholipid membrane bilayers. They may be filled with *gadolinium* to provide a potentially useful contrast agent.

Liver-specific contrast agents

Type of organ-specific agents, which may be further classified into *reticuloendothelial system* (RES) *agents* and *hepatobiliary agents* both of which are taken up by the normal functioning liver.

RES agents are usually *SPIO* or *USPIO* agents (e.g., Endorem, Sinerem etc.). They effect T_2 contrast so that areas of malignancy become conspicuously bright.

Hepatobiliary agents shorten the T_1 of normal liver so that tumors appear dark. These agents are usually gadolinium or manganese based (e.g., Teslascan, Multihance, Eovist).

Loading

The reduction in the *quality factor* of the RF coil when it is positioned on a patient for imaging. Sometimes a loading annulus is used around phantoms to more faithfully simulate the presence of a patient in *quality assurance* tests.

See also *sodium chloride*.

Localizer

Rapid low quality images acquired at the start of an examination and used to subsequently prescribe the diagnostic-quality images. Modern scanners acquire localiser images in all three planes. Other manufacturer specific names for these images include scout images, plan scan, scanogram or even locator.

Logistic regression

A statistical method, were a predictive model is established from the most significant of a given number of input parameters. For example, in classifying benign and malignant disease from dynamic contrast enhanced measurements.

See also *artificial neural networks*.

Long bore

An arbitrary term used to principally describe older closed tunnel systems (especially at high fields) in order to distinguish them from the more modern *short bore* designs.

Long tau inversion recovery

Technique using a very long inversion time (denoted by the Greek letter tau τ), typically 2 s, to null fluid signal with long T_1 relaxation times. It is very useful in the brain to suppress CSF and improve delineation of tumors. Examples include *FLAIR* and Turbo Dark fluid.

See also *short tau inversion recovery*.

Longitudinal magnetization

See *net magnetization*.

Longitudinal plane

The plane parallel to the B_0 field (in the z-direction). It is the plane in which T_1 recovery takes place leading to its alternative name of longitudinal relaxation.

See also *transverse plane*.

Look-Locker

A sequence used to measure T_1 relaxation times. It is based on the *inversion recovery* method but utilizes multiple low flip angle pulses to obtain data in a single TR.

References

Look DC, Locker DR. Time saving in the measurement of NMR and EPR relaxation times. Rev Sci Instrum. 1970;41:250–251

Lorentz force

The force induced on a current carrying conductor in the presence of a magnetic field. The direction of the resulting motion of the conductor is given by Fleming's left hand rule. This can be understood by holding each of the first three fingers of the left hand at right angles to each other and aligning them in the following directions: thuMb = Motion, First finger = Field, seCond finger = current.

In MRI it manifests itself as the *acoustic noise* in the scanner which is produced by the vibrating gradient coils.

Lorentzian shape

The characteristic shape of spectral peaks in MRS (see *linewidth*). It is the *Fourier transformation* of an *exponential* signal.

Low field

Referring to a scanner with a magnetic field strength below 1.0 T.

See also *high field*.

Low gamma (γ) imaging

A phrase used to describe the utilization of MRI for the study of MR visible nuclei with a lower *gyromagnetic ratio* than proton e.g., *sodium*. This is becoming possible thanks to the increase in field strength of many clinical scanners.

Low order phase

The small *phase encoding* steps which correspond to the center of k-space and are responsible for the contrast and signal within the image.

See also *high order phase*.

Low pass filtering

The removal of high frequency components from MRI data, e.g., to achieve image smoothing or blurring. The filter consists of the value 1 below a certain frequency threshold and zero elsewhere. A suitable windowing function (e.g., *Hanning filter*) may be used to reduce ringing artifacts caused by the non-ideal nature of the filtering process.

See also *high pass filtering*.

Lumirem

A contrast agent taken orally and containing iron (*magnetite*) to make the intestine appear dark. Developed by AMAG Pharmaceuticals, it has a generic name of Ferumoxsil (also known as GastroMARK) and a chemical name of AMI-25.

Lung MRI

Traditionally difficult area of MRI which has to overcome three specific complications, namely a low *proton density*, a large *susceptibility artifact* at the air-tissue interface and respiratory motion. The low signal background is actually helpful in certain diseases that demonstrate an increased proton density. Modern r*espiratory gating* methods and motion compensation methods like *radial k-space* continue to increase the efficacy of lung MRI. Ventilation imaging is a growing application owing to the use of hyperpolarised gases (see *hyperpolarised gas imaging*). Other techniques include pulmonary *MRA* and the analysis of respiratory mechanics.

References

Baert AL, Knauth M, Sartor K. MRI of the lung. Berlin: Springer; 2009. ISBN 9783540346180

M

Magic angle effect

An artifact, which appears in parallel fibrous structures, for example ligaments and tendons, at a certain specific angle. The naturally short T_2 values become increased if these fibers are orientated at the magic angle (approximately 54.7° to the direction of B_0), leading to a bright signal. The effect is a phenomenon of dipolar coupling which becomes zero at this precise orientation with a strong magnetic field.

See also *dipole–dipole interactions*.

Magic angle spinning

In vitro technique used to acquire high resolution MRS spectra of solid tissue. Samples are spun at a specific angle (see *magic angle effect*) to make use of the resulting zero coupling effect. This narrows the normally broad spectral peaks of solid material thereby increasing spectral resolution.

Magnet stability

See *stability* and also *field decay*.

Magnetic moment

See *moment*.

Magnetic susceptibility

See *susceptibility*.

Magnetization

The number of magnetic moments produced per unit volume (M) when a material is placed in an external magnetic field (H). It is related to the material's *susceptibility* χ, by:

$$M = \chi H$$

The origin of the magnetization can be due to electrons or the nucleus.

See also *permeability*.

Magnetization transfer

The use of an off-resonance RF pulse to saturate signal from macromolecules (*bound protons*) which creates an entirely new type of image contrast. Quantitative measurements are difficult but are beginning to be applied clinically (see *magnetization transfer ratio*). Appropriate sequences are often denoted MTC for magnetization transfer contrast.

Magnetization transfer ratio

The ratio of the signal measured following the application of a *magnetization transfer* (MT) pulse compared to the signal without the MT pulse. Ratio values are higher in white matter compared to gray matter due to myelin differences. The value is reduced in demyelination.

Magnetization vector

See *net magnetization*.

Magnetite

A naturally occurring magnetic mineral (Ferrous ferric oxide) used in the contrast agent *Lumirem*.

Magnetogyric ratio

Alternative name for the *gyromagnetic ratio*.

Magnetohemodynamic effect

The alteration in the T-wave of an ECG trace due to the presence of the magnetic field of the scanner. It arises from the interaction of the magnetic field on moving charges and the effect increases with field strength.

See also *ECG gating*.

Magnetophosphenes

Flashing lights induced in the eyes due to rapid head motions inside or near to the bore of a high field scanner. It is usually only present in fields of 4.0 T and above.

References

Schenck JF, Dumoulin CL, et al. Human exposure to 4.0 T magnetic field in a whole-body scanner. Med Phys. 1992;19:1089–1098

Magnevist

Commercial name of the gadolinium based *contrast agent* dimeglumine gadopentatate (*Gd-DTPA*) marketed by Schering. The most widely used agent and one with the longest safety record.

Mangafodipir trisodium

The name of the compound used in the contrast agent *Teslascan*.

Manganese

Common relaxation (see *doping*) agent (Mn^{2+}). Its T_2 *relaxivity* is much greater than T_1 relaxivity. Manganese may additionally be used to dope iron oxide particles (see *USPIO*). The high manganese content in some food products make them suitable as an *oral contrast agent*.

Manual shim

The user controlled shimming procedure. This is only ever required if the *auto shim* routine has failed and/or the anatomy is problematic. However, it is usually advisable to perform a manual shim prior to MRS in order to achieve the best spectral quality. The procedure involves iteratively adjusting currents to the shim coils and watching the resulting effect on the water resonance which can be displayed as a FID or as a spectrum (see Fig. 83).

   See also *active shimming* and *FWHM*.

MAS

Abbreviation for *Magic Angle Spinning*.

MAST

Acronym for Motion Artifact Suppression Technique. A flow compensation method relying on *even echo rephasing*.

Matched bandwidth

Name for *variable bandwidth* on Toshiba systems.

Matrix

The number of pixels assigned to each imaging direction. Often the frequency direction is fixed to 256 or 512 but the phase direction can be more variable (e.g., 512 down to 64). A higher image matrix leads to better *spatial resolution* but poorer *SNR*.

Maximum intensity projection

Abbreviated to MIP. This is a 3D reconstruction algorithm which selects the highest pixel intensities along different ray paths cast through the data. It is used in *white blood* MRA to give a 3D visualization of vasculature. Example MIPs are shown in Figs. 57 and 96.

See also *minimum intensity projection*.

Maxwell pair

Design of *gradient coil* consisting of a pair of opposing currents (the opposite of a *Helmholtz pair*). This produces a linear change in magnetic field parallel to their cylindrical axes i.e., the gradient parallel to the direction of B_0 and termed G_z. A diagram of a Maxwell pair is shown in Fig. 43.

See also *Golay coil*.

MDE

Abbreviation for Myocardial Delayed Enhancement. See *delayed contrast enhancement*.

Mean diffusivity

The average of the three eigenvalues determined from the diffusion tensor (see *DTI*). It is equal to the *trace* divided by three.

MEDAL

Acronym for Multi-Echo for Decomposition of Aqua/Lipid. This is the name for the beta version of the *LAVA* sequence.

MEDIC

Acronym for Multi-Echo Data Image Combination. A Siemens sequence with a mixed weighting from the combination of several gradient echoes producing much higher SNR. This is equivalent to the *MERGE* sequence.

MEG

Abbreviation for MagnetoEncephaloGraphy. The measurement of the magnetic field induced by electrical currents in the brain to study brain function. It may be used in conjunction with *fMRI*, offering a very high temporal resolution but lower spatial resolution.

See also *EEG*.

MEMP

An old acronym for the Multi-Echo Multi-Planar sequence. A *multiple-spin echo* sequence from GE that can be used to measure T_2 relaxation times. Unlike *VEMP* the echo spacing is fixed.

MERGE

Acronym from Multiple Echo Reconstructed Gradient Echo. This sequence uses the average signal from multiple gradient-echoes in each TR. A GE sequence that is equivalent to *MEDIC* from Siemens.

MESS

Acronym for Multi-Echo Single-Shot.

Metabolite map

A low spatial resolution image formed from the integration of spectral peak areas from multiple voxel MRSI data. It is usually displayed in a color scale and overlaid onto gray scale anatomical images of higher resolution. The ratio of specific peak areas is often displayed to increase the diagnostic information. This data may be statistically classified in order to highlight abnormal voxels. In so doing the technique has the potential to demonstrate microscopic tumor extensions before they appear on routine images. It has been shown to be particularly useful in prostate and brain (Fig. 53).

See also *MRSI*.

References

Li X, Lu Y, Pirzkall A, McKnight T, Nelson SJ. Analysis of the spatial characteristics of metabolic abnormalities in newly diagnosed glioma patients. J Magn Reson Imaging. 2002;16:229–237

Metallic taste

The unpleasant taste in the mouth, thought to be a stimulation of the palate, which has been anecdotally recorded in magnetic fields of 8.0 T.

Microscopy

The use of dedicated small gradient coils to obtain images with extremely high spatial resolution. Typically refers to

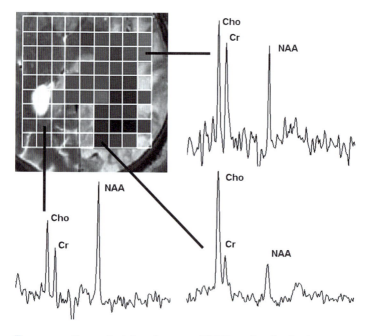

FIGURE 53 Example taken from an MRSI study of a brain tumor. Spectra from three voxels are highlighted with the peaks of choline (cho), creatine (cr) and NAA labeled. The ratio of cho:NAA is calculated on a voxel-by-voxel basis. Abnormally high values are displayed as gray levels and overlaid onto a T_2-weighted image to produce a low resolution *metabolite map*. Liney G. MRI in clinical practice. London: Springer; 2006, p. 71

images with in-plane pixels of 100 μm or smaller. Current 3.0 T clinical scanners are able to produce 200–300 μm images with commercial coils (see *bone imaging*).

Minimum intensity projection

Analogous to the *maximum intensity projection* but instead the algorithm works with the lowest pixel intensities. It is used to display *black blood* angiograms in 3D.

MIP

Acronym for *Maximum Intensity Projection* (pronounced "mip"). It is written as mIP (lowercase m) to indicate the *Minimum Intensity Projection*.

MITR

Abbreviation for Maximum Intensity Time Ratio. A measurement taken from a *signal-time curve* used to display *dynamic contrast enhancement* data. It is similar to *enhancement rate* but it is defined at the maximum percentage enhancement divided by the time taken to reach this value.

Mixing time

The time between the second and third 90° pulse in the *STEAM* spectroscopy sequence, denoted TM. This controls the amount of longitudinal magnetization, which is said to be stored prior to signal detection leading to its alternative name of storage time.

MNS

Abbreviation for Multi-Nuclear Spectroscopy. This describes an examination where imaging is acquired from the proton signal and a spectrum is acquired from a second (non-proton) nucleus. Examples include carbon, fluorine and phosphorus.

See also *dual tune*.

MobiTrak

The name of Philips' *stepping table* MR imaging technique used for *peripheral MRA*.

MOD

Abbreviation for the Magnetic Optical Disc storage medium. See also *OD*.

Moire fringes

Image artifact seen as a result of the *aliasing* of signals with alternating phases. A characteristic zebra-like pattern is superimposed onto the image. Its name comes from an historic term used to describe a type of silk that exhibits a wave pattern. Most commonly observed in 3D gradient echo images at the ends of the volume (Fig. 54).

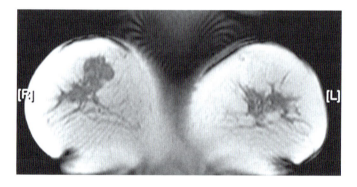

FIGURE 54 Example of *moiré fringes* appearing in this gradient-echo coronal breast image. Liney G. MRI in clinical practice. London: Springer; 2006, p. 50

Molecular imaging

Referring to the use of *nanoparticles* attached to antibodies or proteins in order to provide a contrast agent that specifically targets a site. Currently an active area of research, and examples include iron oxide particles conjugated with herceptin in the study of breast cancer cells.

Molecular tumbling rate

The rate at which a molecule moves, and which governs the T_1 and T_2 relaxation times of a particular tissue. Tumbling rates close to the *Larmor frequency* will produce a short T_1. Tumbling rates both longer and shorter than this increase the T_1 value.

T_2 is roughly proportional to the tumbling rate.

See also *correlation time* and *Bloembergen, Purcell and Pound equation*.

Moment

The small magnetic field associated with spinning nuclear charges. It is usually given the Greek letter mu (μ) and is related to the spin angular momentum of a nucleus (J) by:

$$\mu = \gamma J$$

where γ is the *gyromagnetic ratio* of the nucleus.

Morphological descriptors

The use of subjective or quantitative measurements to describe tumor shape and border. This has proved particularly useful in breast tumor discrimination where a malignant tumor will typically be irregular in shape while a benign tumor appears more round. Some common shape measurements include *circularity*, *convexity, complexity* and *elongatedness* (Fig. 55).

See also *BI-RADS*.

References

Liney GP, Sreenivas M, Gibbs P, Garcia-Alvarez R, Turnbull LW. Breast lesion analysis of shape technique: semiautomated vs manual morphological description. J Magn Reson Imag 2006;23:494–498

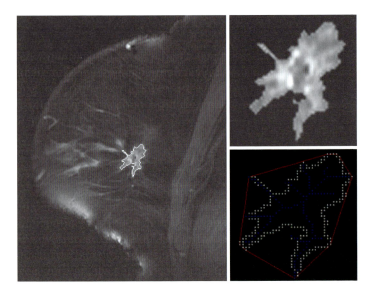

FIGURE 55 (*Left*) A post-contrast breast image demonstrating an irregular region of enhancement. (*Right*) This region is automatically segmented (*top*) and various *morphological descriptors* are calculated (*bottom*). The original border (*white dots*) can be used to measure circularity and complexity. Convexity is determined by fitting straight lines to the shape (shown in *red*). The *blue line* is the end result of a border thinning algorithm used to measure elongatedness

Moses effect

Phenomenon observed in water, which forms two peaks due to its *diamagnetic* properties under certain extreme experimental conditions. This requires a high field and small bore size (e.g., 8.0 T and 5 cm).

MOTSA

Acronym for Multiple Overlapping Thin Section Angiograms. The use of high-resolution 3D MRA scans which sum together to provide a large coverage.

Motion artifact

Increased signal throughout the phase encoding direction due to patient motion.
    See also *Ghosting*.

Motion correction

Hardware or software methods used to reduce the effects of physiological motion. Techniques may be further classed as either prospective or retrospective.
    See also *registration* and *BRACE*.

Moving saturation pulse

A technique whereby a saturation pulse travels at a fixed distance from the slice being acquired thereby optimizing the blood signal. It is implemented under various names such as Walking SAT (GE), Travel SAT (Siemens) or Travel REST (Philips).
    See also *saturation pulses*.

Moving table

Alternative name for *stepping table*.

MPR

Abbreviation of Multi-Planar Reformat.
    See also *reformat*.

MP-RAGE

Acronym for Magnetization Prepared Rapid Acquisition by Gradient Echo. A 3D version of *Turbo FLASH*.

MR compatible

Equipment or device, which is non-ferromagnetic and can therefore be used safely within the scanner (i.e., it is a non-*projectile*). However, it may still cause a large *susceptibility artifact* e.g., *titanium* needles etc.

A simple *deflection angle test* is performed to assess the compatibility of a device.

In the USA a three-level classification of devices is used with appropriate labels to indicate the compatibility. A green square denotes "MR safe," with a red circle and cross through it indicating "MR unsafe." An orange triangle designates "MR conditional," meaning the device or implant is deemed safe only for the stated field strengths.

A useful list concerning the status for a large number of medical implants and devices is provided by the latest Shellock reference book.

References

Shellock FG. Reference manual for magnetic resonance safety, implants and devices. Los Angeles: Biomedical Research Publishing Group; 2005. ISBN: 0974641014

MR cisternography

The use of MRI to image the basal cisterns.

MR dosimetry

The use of MRI for the verification of radiotherapy doses. It involves imaging a radiosensitive gel into which a radiotherapy plan has been delivered. This can then be read out by MRI due to the dose-dependent changes in gel relaxation times. Usually a sample of the gel is first calibrated over a range of doses so that absolute dose in the plan can be measured. Early studies used Fricke gels (where R_1 changed with dose) but these have been replaced by polyacrylamide gels (utilizing R_2 changes). Examples of these include BANG and MAGIC formulations (Fig. 56).

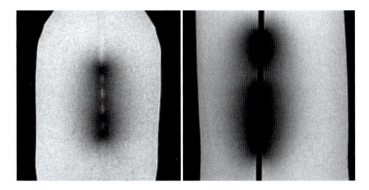

FIGURE 56 *MR dosimetry* examples in high dose-rate brachytherapy. The dark areas on these T_2-weighted images show the dose distributions produced by an iridium wire source which has been inserted into radiosensitive gels

References

Liney GP, Heathcote A, Jenner A, Turnbull LW, Beavis AW. Absolute radiation dose verification using magnetic resonance imaging I: feasibility study. J Radiother Pract. 2003;3:120–127

MR echo

GE's cardiac imaging platform. The name echo refers to the use of high-performance real-time *cine* sequences to replace conventional echocardiography.

MR-GILD

Acronym for MR Gated Intracranial CSF (Liquor) Dynamics. An imaging method using a *bipolar* gradient scheme in order to image the flow of CSF, which is more clearly demonstrated by the subtraction of diastolic and systolic gated images.

MR guided

Referring to any technique in which MR images are used to carry out a procedure. Sometimes denoted MRg and used as a prefix. Examples include a biopsy or placement of a localisation wire in the breast (MR guided biopsy/localization) or treatment of tumors with a heating probe (MR guided focussed ultrasound).

See also *MR thermotherapy* and *interventional device*.

MR mammography

The increasing use of MRI for breast imaging requiring a dedicated *breast coil*. The imaging protocol usually consists of T_1-weighted gradient-echo volumes with and without fat suppression. *Dynamic contrast-enhancement* is also essential and demonstrates a very high sensitivity for breast lesion detection. It has found a specific role in the screening of genetic cancer where young women with dense breasts (X-ray occult lesions) need to be repeatedly scanned. *MR-guided* breast localisation is also on the increase (see *interventional device*). Dedicated sequences exist for both imaging (e.g., *VIBRANT*) and spectroscopy (e.g., *BREASE*, *GRACE*). Example breast images are shown in Figs. 25, 30, and 55.

See also *BI-RADS*, *needle artifacts* and *choline*.

References

Heywang-Kobrunner SH, Beck R. Contrast-enhanced MRI of the breast. Berlin: Springer; 1996

MR myleography

The use of MRI to image the spinal cord, nerve roots and subarachnoid space of the spinal canal using heavily T_2-weighted images.

MR simulator

Mock-up of a real MR scanner used to familiarize claustrophobic patients prior to their examination. More sophisticated simulators also have equipment to reproduce the noise of the scanner. Simulators may also be used to help relax patients prior to *fMRI* in order to achieve better results.

MR thermometry

The use of specific sequences for displaying temperature in vivo usually during some form of thermotherapy (i.e., hypertherapy or cryotherapy). A probe (e.g., *HIFUS*) is used to increase or decrease temperature in a tumor in order to achieve cell death. The progression of this temperature change can be monitored by measurements of T_1, phase, or the resonant frequency shift of water.

References

Matsumoto R, Oshio K, Jolesz FA. Monitoring of laser and freezing-induced ablation in the liver with T_1-weighted MR imaging. J Magn Reson Imaging. 1993;3:770–776

MR thermotherapy

MR-guided treatment of tumors using temperature changes. See also *MR thermometry* and *laser ablation*.

MR oximetry

The use of MRI to non-invasively measure blood oxygen for example using R_2^* maps.

See also *hypoxia*.

MR visible

1. Referring to nuclei with a non-zero spin *quantum number* which are therefore able to produce an MR signal. Common MR visible nuclei include specific isotopes of *hydrogen*, *carbon*, *phosphorus*, and *fluorine*.
2. The description of any foreign material in the patient, which will show up on MR images.

MRA

Abbreviation for MR Angiography. This is the use of MRI to non-invasively image the vascular tree. Many flow related techniques are used such as time-of-flight (*TOF*) and *phase-contrast* and also increasingly *contrast-enhanced MRA*. Non-contrast techniques involve sensitizing the imaging sequence to the flow of blood with resulting signal changes that are usually dependent on velocity or direction. Some techniques are additionally able to separate arteries from veins.

See also *peripheral MRA* and *maximum intensity projection*.

MRE

Abbreviation for MR Elastography. Emerging technique which images the propagation of mechanically produced shear waves through tissue in order to measure their stiffness. Results are displayed as a parameter map called an *elastogram*.

MRCP

Abbreviation for MR CholangioPancreatography. This refers to the use of MRI for non-invasive imaging of the hepatobilliary system (bile ducts, pancreas and liver). Sequences that are heavily T_2-weighted are used to show fluid within ducts (Fig. 57).

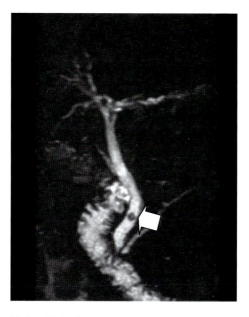

FIGURE 57 This *MRCP* image displayed as a MIP demonstrates a bile duct stone. Liney G. MRI in clinical practice. London: Springer; 2006, p. 91

MRS

Abbreviation for Magnetic Resonance Spectroscopy. The measurement and display of *chemical shift* information from a small volume. Results are displayed in the form of a spectrum of peak amplitudes at specific frequencies which are used to identify the metabolites present in the sample.

Proton is the most widely studied nucleus requiring *water suppression* in order to visualize much smaller concentrated resonances. This gives the technique an inherently poor signal-to-noise ratio (*SNR*) and reduces the resolution compared to imaging. Other nuclei studied with MRS include *phosphorus*, *carbon*, *sodium* and *fluorine*.

MRS may be acquired as either a *single-voxel* or *multi-voxel* technique. Due to the requirement for the preservation of inherent frequency differences, localisation of the signal is achieved without frequency encoding. Common methods include *PRESS* and *STEAM*.

Multi-voxel acquisitions are more commonly referred to as MRS imaging (*MRSI*).

References

Salibi N, Brown MA. Clinical MR spectroscopy: first principles. New York: Wiley; 1998. ISBN: 047118280X

MRSI

Abbreviation for MR Spectroscopic Imaging. A 2D or 3D *MRS* technique in which a volume is localized and then subdivided into smaller contiguous voxels using phase encoding (see *multi-voxel*). The spatial resolution of each voxel is typically limited to around 1 cm^3 (for proton) but this can be reduced to as little as 0.2 cm^3 if a *surface coil* is used. The resulting data is often turned into a *metabolite map* (Fig. 58).

MS-325

The chemical name for the *blood pool agent* known commercially as *AngioMARK*.

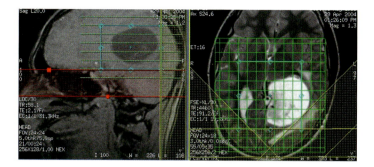

FIGURE 58 Graphical prescription of an *MRSI* examination. The volume of interest (*blue*) is positioned using images previously acquired as part of the examination together with the display of a grid (*green*) indicating the location of the spectroscopy voxels. Saturation bands (*red and yellow*) may also be appropriately positioned to reduce signal contamination

MSE

Abbreviation of *Multiple Spin-Echo*.

MSK imaging

Abbreviation for *MusculoSKeletal imaging*.

mSENSE

Abbreviation for modified *SENSE*.

mT/m

The units of gradient strength. 10 mT/m is equivalent to 1 G cm^{-1}. Modern scanners have peak amplitudes of up to 50 mT m^{-1}.

MT

Abbreviation for *Magnetization Transfer*.

MTF

Abbreviation for Modulation Transfer Function. A Quantitative measure of spatial resolution, which is more reliable than visualizing signal variations across bar patterns. Instead, a pixel profile is taken across an angled block, to give an edge response function. The derivative of this gives the line spread function. The *Fourier transformation* of the line spread function then gives the MTF which provides information at all spatial frequencies.

See also *spatial resolution*.

References

Judy PF. The line spread function and modulation transfer function of a computed tomography scanner. Med Phys. 1976;3:233–236

MTT

Abbreviation for Mean Transit Time.
See also *transit time*.

MU

Greek letter (μ) used to denote magnetic *moment*, *permeability* and also to express units of 10^{-6} (or micro).

Multi-echo

Referring to any sequence acquiring more than one echo in a single repetition time (*TR*) e.g., *multiple spin-echo* or *FSE*.

Multi-nuclear spectroscopy

See *MNS*.

Multi-planar

Referring to the multiple slice 2D imaging capability of MRI.

See also *reformat*.

Multi-slab

Referring to the acquisition of more than one 3D volume (or slab). For example in *time-of-flight* (TOF) techniques, the thickness of a volume is limited due to saturation effects and it may be advantageous to acquire multi-slabs. Also referred to as multi-chunk.

Multi-slice

The acquisition of more than one slice per repetition time by utilizing the *dead time* in a sequence to acquire other slices.

Multi-voxel

An MRS acquisition from multiple contiguous voxels rather than a single-voxel. These voxels can be acquired in a line, in a single 2D grid or covering several slices (3D). This has the advantage of measuring chemical information from several simultaneous regions-of-interest across an image although the spatial resolution of each voxel is still limited (see *voxel bleeding*).

See also *MRSI*.

MultiHance

Commercial name for a contrast agent (developed by Bracco), which binds weakly and reversibly to blood protein albumin. This improves its relaxivity and usefulness as a *blood pool agent*. Its generic name is Godobenate dimeglumine and its chemical name is Gd-BOPTA.

Multi-channel

An RF coil *array* in which the separate coil elements have their own independent receiver components (or channels). This improves signal-to-noise ratio (*SNR*) and enables signal from the coils to be combined in a useful way for example in *parallel imaging*. Typical modern systems have between 8 and 32 channels.

Multiple spin-echo

A spin echo sequence where more than one echo is acquired (usually four or more). Unlike the fast spin echo (*FSE*) sequence, these echoes have the same phase encoding so that multiple separate images are produced. It can be used to measure T_2 relaxation time.

See also *CPMG*.

Multi-phase

Description of a sequence in which each slice is acquired more than once to produce a *dynamic* acquisition. It is denoted as MP on *DICOM* images.

Multi-shot

Term used to describe an ultra-fast imaging sequence that does not acquire all of k-space in a single repetition time (unlike *single-shot*), and therefore requires more than one acquisition.

See also *EPI*.

MULTIVANE

Name for Philips version of their motion correction technique by using a *radial k-space* acquisition.

See also *k-space trajectory* and *PROPELLER*.

Musculoskeletal imaging

The use of MRI in the diagnosis of joint disease, bone disease and assessment of masses in soft-tissue and bone. Good quality off-center imaging of the shoulder is now possible with improvements in B_0 homogeneity. Hand and wrist imaging is optimized with dedicated wrist coils and higher field systems. Open or wide bore systems permit *kinematic imaging* of the knee (Fig. 59).

See also *bone imaging* and *delayed contrast enhancement*.

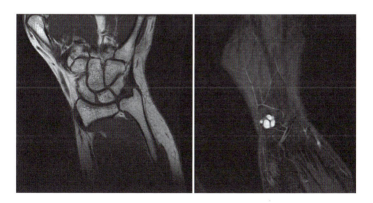

FIGURE 59 Examples of *musculoskeletal imaging* in the wrist. (*Left*) A T_1-weighted image shows trabecular detail and (*right*) a ganglion can be seen in this fat suppressed image

M_x, M_y, M_z

Notation used for the transverse (M_x, M_y) and longitudinal (M_z) components of the *net magnetization* (M_0).

Myocardial tagging

See *spin tagging*.

Myo-inositol

A metabolite occurring in ^1H MRS of the brain at 3.56 and 4.06 ppm. Its short T_2 relaxation time means that a short TE acquisition is required to see it.

N

NAA

Abbreviation for N-Acetyl Aspartate. Important metabolite seen in proton MRS of the brain, which is evident in neuronal tissue but reduced in brain tumors (see Fig. 53). It is often used in conjunction with *choline* as a marker of tumor and has a resonance at 2.01 and 2.6 ppm (Fig. 60).

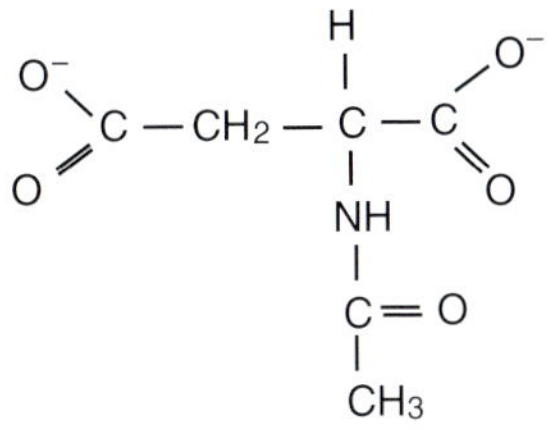

FIGURE 60 The chemical structure of *NAA*

NAAG

Abbreviation for N-Acetyl AspartylGlutamic acid. Provides a small contribution to the NAA peak seen in proton MRS.

Nanoparticles

Designation of particles of between 1 and 100 nm in size. In MRI their interest is in providing contrast agents which may be distributed further than conventional agents and provide increased *relaxivity* for a given dose due to their small size. *USPIO* type agents can be classed as nanoparticles but the term is often used to describe even smaller agents that

215

are currently under development and not yet for clinical use. Examples include gadolinium-doped gold particles, Gd-DTDTPA, *liposomes*, and monocrystalline iron oxide nanoparticles (MIONs).

See also *molecular imaging*.

NATIVE

Name of the non contrast enhanced *MRA* sequence from Siemens. Similar sequences include TRANCE (Philips), InHance (GE), FBI/CIA (Toshiba) and VASC (Hitachi).

The term native is also used generally to refer to tissue relaxation times before they have been affected by a contrast agent.

NAV

1. *DICOM* notation for NAVigator echo.
2. Abbreviation for Number of Averages.

See also *averaging* and *NEX*.

Navigator echo

A *respiratory gating* method, which involves monitoring the signal changes in the direction of motion. Typically the user prescribes a small region of interest across a boundary, for example over the diaphragm, and the imaging is synchronized according to the signal change from this area. Some systems perform a learning phase to automatically adjust for different breathing patterns.

NbTi

Chemical formula for the alloy of *Niobium-titanium*.

Needle artifacts

Specific type of *susceptibility artifact* caused by an *MR compatible* needle which may be used in an *MR guided* biopsy or localisation. The extent and characteristic of the artifact depends on the trajectory of the needle in relation to the main magnetic field, the needle material and the imaging sequence used.

Artifacts are observed along the length of the needle when it is perpendicular to B_o but a *blooming ball* artifact is seen at the end of the needle when it is parallel to B_o. Higher field strengths will produce larger effects. Gradient-echo based sequences are inherently prone to artifacts and these can be reduced by using spin-echo sequences. The nature of the material used for the needle is also important (see *susceptibility*).

An understanding of the directional nature of these susceptibility artifacts is important in other settings, for example careful positioning in orthopedic imaging may reduce the effects of screws on the images.

References

Lewin JS, Duerk JL, Jain VR, et al. Needle localization in MR-guided biopsy and aspiration: effects of field strength, sequence design, and magnetic orientation. AJR Am J Roentgenol. 1996;166:9

NEMA

Acronym for the National Electrical Manufactures Association. See *DICOM*.

Net magnetization

The summation of all the individual magnetic moments in a sample. The net magnetization is denoted M_0 and its use simplifies the description of the MRI phenomenon. Outside of the scanner, i.e., in no external magnetic field, this value is zero. In the presence of a magnetic field, a small finite value aligned with the direction of B_0, is established and called the longitudinal magnetization. After an excitation pulse this component is reduced to zero and there is a full transverse component. The behavior of the net magnetization is shown in Fig. 78.

Neutron

A particle in the nucleus of atoms (a *nucleon*), which has zero charge and a slightly different mass to a *proton* $(1.675 \times 10^{-27}$ kg$)$.

NEX

Acronym for Number of EXcitations. A GE term for signal *averaging*. Signal-to-noise is proportional to the square root of NEX. May also be termed *NSA*, or simply the number of averages.

Nickel

Common relaxation (*doping*) agent (Ni^{2+}). Its T_1 and T_2 *relaxivity* values are similar, and approximately the same as copper.

Niobium-titanium

An alloy which becomes superconducting below $-269°C$ and is used in the construction of a *superconducting magnet*.

Nitrogen

The MR visible isotope of nitrogen (^{15}N) has a low sensitivity but this can be improved through the process of *hyperpolarisation*.

NMR

Abbreviation for Nuclear Magnetic Resonance, the historic term for MRI. The word "nuclear" was dropped in the 1980s because of connotations with nuclear power. The term NMR is now usually reserved for spectroscopy on high field laboratory research systems.

2D NMR refers to correlation spectroscopy and examples include *COSY* and *NOESY* (Fig. 61).

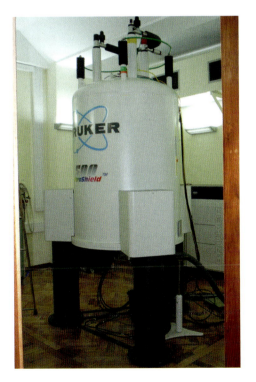

FIGURE 61   A 500 MHz (11.7 T) Bruker *NMR* system which was used to produce the COSY spectrum shown in Fig. 19. Courtesy of Mark Lorch (University of Hull)

NOE

Abbreviation for *Nuclear Overhauser Effect*.

NOESY

Abbreviation for Nuclear Overhauser Effect Spectroscopy. A type of 2D NMR experiment where information is generated concerning the cross-relaxation of spins as opposed to J-coupling in *COSY*. Cross peaks indicate that spins at those frequencies are close in space.

No phase wrap

A scanner option which permits imaging with a small field-of-view (FOV) without aliasing in the phase direction. The scanner acquires a larger FOV than prescribed and increases the image matrix to maintain resolution, but only the desired FOV is displayed. The number of signal averages may also be reduced to improve efficiency. It is also known as anti-aliasing or fold-over suppression.

See also *phase wrap*.

Noise

The random signal contribution to the image. The main source of this signal is from thermal motion within the patient. Image noise is detected from the entire sensitive volume of the RF coil, which is the reason that coil sizes are constrained to the minimum required for the anatomy being imaged. The effect of noise may be further reduced by employing signal *averaging*.

See also *signal* and *SNR*.

Normal mode

A designated operational level of the scanner where the patient should experience no effects.

See also *bio-effects*, *controlled mode*, *research mode* and *safety limits*.

Normalization filter

An image filter used as a *coil uniformity correction*.

NP

DICOM notation for No Phase wrap.

NSA

Abbreviation used by Philips for Number of Signal Averages.
See also *NEX*.

Nu

Greek letter (υ) used to denote frequency.

Nuclear overhauser effect

The enhancement of signal from one nuclei by an adjacent resonance. A common example of the application of this technique is in ^{13}C spectroscopy, where the carbon spectrum of a molecule is improved by interacting with a coupled ^{1}H resonance.

See also *NOESY*.

Nucleon

An elementary atomic particle within the nucleus (i.e., a neutron or proton).

Null point

The point following an *inversion pulse* when the recovering magnetization has a zero longitudinal component (M_z). The null point (TI_{null}) for a particular tissue is related to its T_1 relaxation time and can be determined from the *inversion recovery* signal equation as:

$$S(TI_{null}) = \left[1 - 2\exp(-TI_{null}/T_1)\right] = 0$$

Which can solved to give:

$$TI_{null} = Ln(2) \times T_1$$

The *inversion time* can be set to an appropriate null point value to produce either fat or water suppression. The null point for fat at 1.5 T is approximately 200 ms and the corresponding value for water is around 2 s.

See also *STIR*, *inversion recovery* and *TI*.

Nutation

A slight irregular motion of a body undergoing an otherwise symmetrical rotation. In MRI it can be used to describe the movement of a spin away from its precessional motion when applying an *excitation pulse*. The term nutation angle can be used interchangeably for flip angle although this is not now commonly used.

Nyquist frequency

The specific sampling rate at which frequency aliasing is avoided. Signals at higher frequencies than the sampling rate will be attributed as an erroneously lower frequency. To avoid this, the sampling rate must be twice the highest detected frequency.

See also *frequency wrap*.

Nyquist ghosting

A specific instance of *ghosting* that is observed at half the field-of-view. It is commonly seen in *EPI* due to images being acquired with both positive and negative gradients, meaning k-space is filled in opposite directions. Line-to-line variations in the data acquisition become Fourier transformed into these distinctive ghosts (Fig. 62).

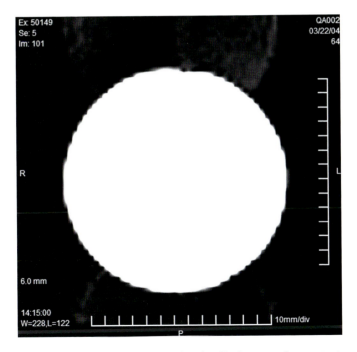

FIGURE 62 This EPI image of a head coil phantom demonstrates *nyquist ghosting*

O

Occupational exposure

A european directive (2004/40/EC) regarding the exposure of workers to electromagnetic fields was set for introduction in 2004. This potential legislation would have imposed serious restrictions on working practices in MRI and its introduction has been delayed until 2012 pending a review of more recent findings.

See also *safety limits*.

Oblique

A non-orthogonal scan plane created by the combination of at least two of the imaging gradients in order to acquire a slice in an angled orientation.

See also *axial*, *coronal*, *sagittal* and *double oblique*.

OD

Abbreviation for Optical Disc. Image archiving medium, which typically holds 2.3 GB of storage. Other common media include *DAT* and *CD*.

Off-center FOV

Imaging where the center of the image has to be necessarily positioned away from the isocenter for example in shoulder imaging. This has the potential for loss of image quality due to the B_0 homogeneity being poorer further away from the isocenter. This is also known as shift offset or FOV offset on some systems.

See also B_0 *inhomogeneity* and *DSV*.

Off-resonance

Referring to the use of an RF excitation pulse with a center frequency other than that of water, for example fat, *silicon* or in *magnetization transfer* imaging.

Omega

Greek letter (ω) used to denote *angular frequency*.
    See also *radians*.

Omniscan

Trade name of a *gadolinium* based contrast agent from Winthrop Laboratories. It is a non-ionic agent chelated to DTPA-bis-methyl-amide (Gd-DTPA-BMA) and referred to as gadodiamide.
    See also *Gd-DTPA*.

OOPS

Acronym for Out Of Phase Scanning. A technique where images are deliberately acquired with fat and water out of phase (using TE=2.1 ms at 1.5 T). This leads to improved visualization in certain instances for example reduced periorbital fat in MRA.
    See also *chemical shift ("of the second kind")*, *DIXON* and *fat water in-phase*.

Open scanner

The design of a magnet with a more open configuration compared to conventional closed (tunnel) systems. This helps to reduce the incidence of *claustrophobia* and also may allow minor interventional procedures to be performed during imaging. Open scanners can have a horizontal bore but the majority have a *vertical bore* design. Usually these scanners have *low field* strength and a greater B_0 *inhomogeneity* compared to standard closed configurations (typically <5 ppm for 40 cm *DSV*). The majority of these scanners use a *permanent magnet* or *resistive magnet* although some higher field systems are superconducting.

Common types of open scanner are described as having a *double donut* or *pillar* design. Some vertical systems use the extra efficiency provided by *solenoid* RF coils to improve signal to that equivalent to a higher field system (termed "high field open") e.g., Philips Panorama HFO 1.0 T which provides "1.5 T" image quality.

See also *interventional device* and *wide bore*.

Optical pumping

A method of providing *hyperpolarised gas imaging*. In a magnetic field, laser light is used to polarize electrons of rubidium atoms and this is transferred to other nuclei by collisions. It has become more practical due to the development of high powered lasers.

Optical RF

The use of fiber optic connections in the RF receiver coils instead of copper wiring. This eliminates electrical noise and improves signal detection. An example is GE's OpTix system which claims to improve signal-to-noise ratio (SNR) by 27%.

OptiMARK

Commercial name for the gadolinium-based contrast agent known as gadoversetamide and developed by Mallinckrodt. It has a chemical name of *Gd-DTPA*-BMEA (where BMEA is bismethoxyethylamide).

Optimized bandwidth

Name for *variable bandwidth* on Siemens systems.

Oral contrast agent

An MR contrast agent which is administered orally in order to image the gastrointestinal tract. Commercial examples include *Lumirem*. Natural food products can also be used (e.g., blueberry juice and green tea) due to their high *manganese* content. Another example includes perflubron (see *perflurocarbon*).

See also *contrast agents*.

Orbit X-ray

A *screening* X-ray of the eyes taken as a safety precaution prior to the MRI examination if there are any concerns with regards to the patient history e.g., previous metal work, shrapnel injury (Fig. 63).

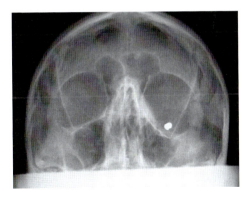

FIGURE 63 An *orbit X-ray* taken as part of patient screening reveals this air-gun pellet. Liney G. MRI in clinical practice. London: Springer; 2006, p. 32

Orientation

For a patient in the head first-supine position the x,y and z directions are defined as shown in Fig. 64.

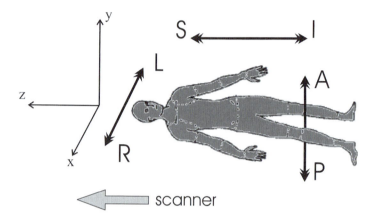

FIGURE 64 Diagram illustrating the *orientation* convention used in MRI. The directions of superior, inferior, anterior, posterior, left and right are defined in terms of the patient position and these are shown in relation to the fixed axes of the scanner

Out-of-phase image

An image acquired at a specific echo time so that the water and fat signal are exactly out of phase. An example is shown in Fig. 10.

See also *chemical shift* (*"of the second kind"*) and *fat-water in-phase.*

Outer k-space

Referring to the edges of k-space, which correspond to image data obtained using the higher phase encoding gradients and contain the high spatial frequency information (image detail).

Outer volume fat suppression

A fat suppression method, which places *saturation bands* outside the volume of interest. It is useful in MRS to reduce contamination from signal outside of the voxels (see Fig. 58).

See also *VSS*.

Overlay

Areas of an image that are highlighted, usually in color, to signify some property or function of that image or the fusion of some secondary image. Examples include the activation areas in *fMRI* or areas of large contrast uptake in a *dynamic contrast enhancement* study. The appearance of the overlay can be set by its *transparency*, leaving the underlying pixel data unaltered. In some instances the highlighted pixels are hard-coded into the image and replace those pixel values (see "*burnt in*" *pixels*).

Over-ranging

The washed-out appearance of an image when the signal extends beyond the receiver range and the data is truncated. Also known as data clipping, overflow or *halo artifact*. It may occur as a result of the dynamic range not being set properly during the *pre-scan*. In certain situations e.g., during a dynamic contrast enhanced study, the signal received may become higher than expected during the course of the scan.

See also *EDR*.

Oversampling

The prevention of aliasing in the frequency direction by increasing the number of measured data points (see *nyquist frequency*). In most scanners frequency oversampling is always on.

See also *phase wrap* and *frequency wrap*.

Oxford instruments

A company based in England selling a wide range of super-conducting magnets including new *cryogen free* magnets.

Oxygen

The naturally abundant *isotope* of oxygen (^{16}O) is not MR visible but the less abundant ^{17}O has a non-zero spin *quantum number* ($I = 5/2$).

Molecular oxygen is weakly paramagnetic and its effect can be observed when it is dissolved in the blood, typically leading to 10% reduction in blood T_1 values. This property can be used in *ventilation imaging* when *carbogen* or 100% oxygen is inhaled and a comparison is made with normal air-ventilated images.

P

PACE

Acronym for Prospective Acquisition CorrEction. A sequence from Siemens utilizing a *navigator echo* to monitor lung displacement and reduce motion artifacts by accepting images acquired within a certain displacement. The technique be applied in one to three dimensions.

Pacemakers

Electronic devices which are used to regulate a patient's heart rate (and also include *ICDs*). Their functionality is altered in the presence of a strong magnetic field and as such they constitute an absolute contraindication. Other safety considerations include the potential for *RF heating* of the leads. It is thought that around a dozen deaths may have been attributable to the inadvertent scanning of pacemakers.

As a safety precaution, members of the public are precluded from encroaching the *five gauss line*.

In future, certain modern pacemakers may overcome this compatibility issue although strict scanning procedures will have to be adopted.

See also *fringe field* and *contraindications*.

PACS

Acronym for Picture Archiving Communication System. Term used to describe the control of archival and transfer of digital images across hospital networks.

Palatal stimulation

The stimulation of nerves of the palate due to rapid movements of the head inside a high field scanner.

See also *metallic taste*.

Paradigm

Term used in functional MRI (*fMRI*) to describe the activation protocol. In its basic form this involves a repetition of a
specific stimulus (known as the "ON" period) followed by a
period of control or rest where the stimulus is not present
(known as "OFF"). The stimulus is related to the area of
brain being examined. A commonly used paradigm is *finger
tapping* in order to activate the primary motor cortex. Many
other more complicated paradigms have been used to study
language, visual and sensory functioning.

See also *box car*, *event related*, *goggles*, *Wada test* and *silent
word generation*.

Paradoxical enhancement

Referring to any flow-related effect resulting in bright signal
rather than signal voids e.g., *in-flow enhancement*.

Parahydrogen

A specific state of molecular hydrogen where the nuclei spins
are orientated so that their moments cancel. It is used in
parahydrogen-induced polarization.

Parahydrogen-induced polarization

A specific method of nuclear *hyperpolarization.* A substance of low MR sensitivity (e.g., ^{13}C) is hydrogenated with

parahydrogen so that the spin ordering of the parahydrogen is converted to nuclear polarization. The material is prepared as a pharmaceutical and injected into the blood to be imaged.

See also *dynamic nuclear polarization* and *hyperpolarized gas imaging*.

References

Goldman M, et al. Hyperpolarization of ^{13}C through order transfer from parahydrogen: a new contrast agent for MRI. Magn Reson Imaging. 2005;23:153–157

Parallel imaging

A technique used to speed up scan times by replacing some of the phase encoding steps with coil sensitivity profiles from *multi-channel* RF coils. The strength of signal from one coil with respect to another is an alternative way of providing localisation of the signal. The missing lines of k-space data are reconstructed from combinations of the separate coil signals. Reconstruction can occur in either k-space or by unwrapping signals in image space. The speed-up factor is given by the number of phase encoding lines that have been omitted. This can theoretically be equal to the number of separate coils used but is usually limited to between 2 and 4. The technique can be thought of in terms of substituting part of the "gradient encoding" with "coil encoding." However, there is a trade-off in terms of decreased SNR which is given by:

$$SNR' = SNR / g \sqrt{R}$$

where g is the geometry factor (≥ 1), which is a coil-specific parameter that has been shown to vary with the reduction factor (R) used.

Parallel imaging is increasingly used to speed-up sequences without associated stimulation problems (see *peripheral nerve stimulation*). It is also useful at high field to overcome susceptibility artifacts and for high *SAR* sequences.

Several implementations exist based on either the k-space (SMASH, GRAPPA) or the image-based approach to reconstruction (SENSE, ASSET).

References

Carlson JW, Minemura T. Imaging time reduction through multiple receiver coil data acquisition and image reconstruction. Magn Reson Med. 1993;29:681–687

Paramagnetic

Material with a positive magnetic susceptibility i.e., when placed in a magnetic field an internal field is induced in the direction of this field. It is a property of material with unpaired electrons e.g., *gadolinium* ions (Gd^{3+}) which is a common constituent of many *contrast agents*.

See also *diamagnetic* and *ferromagnetic*.

Parameter map

A post-processed image that demonstrates some quantitative measurement on a pixel-by-pixel basis. Examples include, a T_2 *map* calculated from several T_2-weighted images or a *positive enhancement integral* from *dynamic contrast enhancement* data. Usually the image is displayed with a color scale rather than *grayscale* to distinguish it from the *raw data*. Examples of parameter maps are shown in Figs. 1, 15, 33, 67, 75, and 93.

Partial echo

The utilization of a partially sampled signal echo in order to reduce scan time. Usually the second half of the echo is sampled and this is equivalent to acquiring only the right hand side of k-space. This may also be called asymmetric, fractional or half echo or more explicitly as partial read Fourier.

Partial flip

The use of a less than 90° *flip angle* for signal excitation. In certain situations (e.g., TR>>T$_1$) the signal is optimized by using a small flip angle (see *Ernst angle*). This arises from the mathematical rule that for small angles the cosine of the angle is approximately equal to 1. A transverse component of magnetization may still be generated (given by M$_0$sinα) while the longitudinal component remains practically unchanged (M$_0$cos$\alpha \approx$ M$_0$). This means signal can recover sufficiently even with a short repetition time.

See also *gradient-echo*.

Partial Fourier

A method of reducing imaging time by acquiring only a fraction of the phase encoding steps. Partial Fourier or more specifically partial phase Fourier, usually refers to the acquisition of the bottom half of k-space rather than the term *partial k-space*, which is less specific. In practice slightly more than half of the lines of k-space are acquired, with the missing data subsequently filled-in due to *conjugate symmetry*.

Partial Fourier is also known as halfscan, half Fourier, partial or fractional NEX and 1/2 NEX. Other fractions of k-space may also be acquired for example three-quarters, often referred to as 3/4 NEX imaging.

Partial k-space

General term used to describe an imaging technique where only part of the k-space data is acquired in order to speed up imaging time. Conventionally lines of k-space are filled left-to-right by frequency encoding and bottom-to-top by incremental phase encoding per TR. In *partial echo* only the right half of k-space is acquired. In *partial Fourier*, only the bottom half of k-space is collected. Missing data is filled in by taking advantage of the *conjugate symmetry* properties of k-space.

See also *key-hole imaging*.

Partial NEX

See *Partial Fourier*.

Partial saturation

The condition that arises when a scan is acquired with a sufficiently short repetition time (TR) so that complete T_1 recovery of the signal is not achieved.

Partial volume

The effect of reduced signal and contrast when spatial resolution is large compared to the structure being studied. For example when pixel size is coarse or thick slices are used, adjacent regions with different signal intensities contribute to on overall average pixel intensity value.

Parts per million

Usually abbreviated to *PPM*.

PASADENA

Acronym for Para And Synthesis Allows Dramatically Enhanced Nuclear Alignment. The original term for *parahydrogen induced polarization*.

PASL

Abbreviation for Pulsed *Arterial Spin Labeling*.

Passive shielding

Type of magnet shielding making use of steel placed at certain parts of the magnet as opposed to *active shielding*.

See also *fringe field*.

Passive shimming

The use of ferromagnetic plates positioned inside the windings of the magnet to improve the homogeneity of the B_0 field.

See also *shim* and *active shimming*.

Patient right

Referring to the conventional radiological presentation of images such that the patient's right side is displayed on the left of axial and coronal images for head-first supine positioning (see Fig. 3 and 18).

See also *orientation*.

Patient table

Part of the scanner on which the patient is positioned and landmarked. The table top then moves the patient into the magnet *isocenter*. In some scanners the table may be detachable for ease of transfer of some ambulant patients. A flat table top may also be used in *radiotherapy planning*.

Patient weight

The value for the patient weight is entered prior to scanning to correctly calculate and monitor the *SAR* level caused by *RF heating*. The patient table will also have an operational weight limit.

PBSG

Acronym for Phase Balanced *SARGE*.

PC

Abbreviation of *Phase Contrast*.

PD

Abbreviation for *Proton-Density*.

Peak amplitude

The maximum signal measured at a specific resonant frequency in the MR *spectrum*.

Peak area

The integrated area under a peak in the MR *spectrum*, which is proportional to the number of spins at that resonant frequency. The integration can be performed between manually chosen frequency limits. Alternatively the areas can be obtained by fitting the spectrum to a suitable model.

See also *LC model*.

Peak area ratios

Method of quantifying metabolite concentrations in MRS by normalizing the peak area relative to some other peak. The denominator should be a constant signal used as a reference or another signal that changes in the opposite way in order to improve the sensitivity of the measurement. Usually internal peak areas are measured but external reference samples are also used (see *GRACE*).

See also *absolute peak quantification*.

PEAR

Philips technique for *respiratory gating* which is an acronym of Phase Encoded Artifact Reduction. It utilizes real-time adjustment of k-space filling, which is dependent on the position of the diaphragm.

Perflurocarbon

A chemically inert compound formed by replacing the hydrogen atoms in hydrocarbons with fluorine atoms. The material can be used to fill an inflatable type *endorectal coil* which reduces the *susceptibility* artifact compared to using air.

Perflubron is a perflurocarbon that has been used as a gastrointestinal contrast agent which works by appearing dark due to the lack of proton signal. Perflurocarbons may even be imaged directly using ^{19}F MRI (see *fluorine*) although this is still in its infancy.

Perfusion

Blood flow at the capillary level, or more specifically the flow rate per unit of tissue mass.

Perfusion imaging

Referring to a variety of techniques for imaging and monitoring tissue *perfusion*. These can be subdivided into *arterial spin labeling* (or ASL) and *dynamic susceptibility contrast* methods.

Arterial spin labeling works by magnetically labeling spins in a number of ways depending on the actual sequence.

Dynamic susceptibility contrast uses a contrast agent and T_2^* images to examine tissue perfusion via susceptibility effects as the agent traverses through capillaries. Signal is seen to decrease in the perfused region and blood volume and flow can be mathematically described. Usually an *arterial input function* is also required.

Perfusion imaging is useful in cancer and also in stroke, where *diffusion* may overestimate the ischemic area.

See also *cerebral blood flow (volume)*.

References

Calamante F, Thomas DL, Pell GS, et al. Measuring cerebral blood flow using magnetic resonance imaging techniques. J Cereb Blood Flow Metab. 1999;19:701–735

Peripheral enhancement

See *rim enhancement*.

Peripheral MRA

A specific application of MR angiography (see *MRA*) most commonly performed with contrast enhancement to image the vessels of the arms or legs. Peripheral MRA in the legs requires *stepping table* scans, dedicated RF coils and double doses of contrast to improve the signal (Fig. 65).

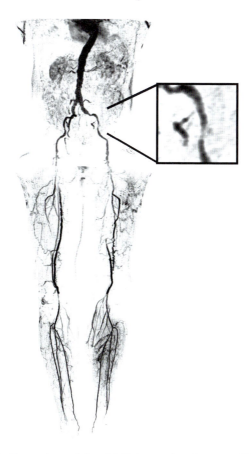

FIGURE 65 Example *peripheral MRA* covering the aorto-illiac arteries down to the tibial arteries. Liney G. MRI in clinical practice. London: Springer; 2006, p. 114

Peripheral nerve stimulation

Abbreviated to PNS. A harmless but sometimes unpleasant involuntary effect usually experienced in the fingers or nose. It is induced by rapid gradient switching which is required in order to acquire scans as quickly as possible. PNS typically occurs around $60\,\mathrm{T\,s^{-1}}$ but is dependant on gradient *rise times*. The threshold for nerve stimulation in humans has been modeled and a useful expression, which fits experimental data is given by:

$$\frac{dB}{dt} = 54\left(1+\left(\frac{132}{t}\right)\right)$$

where t is the rise time in μs.

Potentially fatal cardiac stimulation occurs well above this threshold (for rise times <1 ms). *Zoom gradients* reduce the effect even at high switching rates by reducing the extent of the gradient.

The desire to further reduce imaging time without the risk of stimulation has lead to the development of a technique called *parallel imaging.*

See also *db/dt.*

References

Reilly JP. Principles of nerve and heart excitation by time-varying magnetic fields. Ann NY Acad Sci. 1992;649:96–117

Peripheral pulse gating

A particular *gating* method using a light transducer (a *photoplethysmograph*) attached to the fingertip to detect pulse rate. At high fields it is more reliable than *ECG gating*.

See also *PQRST wave.*

Peristaltic motion

Semi-random physiological motion of the intestine which can cause motion artifacts in abdominal imaging. This may be reduced by administering an anti-peristaltic agent e.g., buscopan or fasting for 4 h prior to the scan.

Permanent magnet

A type of scanner constructed from ferromagnetic material in which a field has been established during manufacture. They tend to be very heavy but have low running costs and achieve fields of around 0.2–0.3 T. Early types used iron–cobalt alloys but modern versions use rare alloys such as samarium cobalt and neodymium iron boron, which reduces the weight.

See also *superconducting magnet* and *resistive magnet*.

Permeability

A constant denoted by the Greek letter mu (μ) that describes magnetic susceptibility.

The permeability of a material relates the induced magnetic field (B) created within it by an externally applied field (H):

$$B = \mu H$$

and

$$\mu = \mu_0 (1 + \chi)$$

where μ_0 is the permeability in a vacuum (so called "permeability of free space") and χ is the *susceptibility*. Relative permeability μ_r is defined as the ratio μ/μ_0 (equal to $1+\chi$). μ_0 is equal to $4\pi \times 10^{-7}$ N A^{-2}.

Permeability is the magnetic analog to *permittivity*.

Permittivity

A constant denoted by the Greek letter epsilon (ε) that describes the electric susceptibility of a material. It is also referred to as the dielectric constant.

See also *dielectric effect*.

PERRM

Acronym for Phase Encode Reordering to Reduce Motion. A *respiratory gating* technique from Hitachi.

Perspex

A common type of plastic used in the construction of MRI phantoms as its magnetic *susceptibility* is similar to that of water.

PET

Acronym for Positron Emission Tomography. It is a specific nuclear medicine technique utilizing high energy positron emitting nuclides, which are detected using coincidence detectors. Often used in functional studies and compared to *fMRI* data, but with disadvantages of poorer spatial resolution and ionizing radiation.

Hybrid MRI-PET systems with the detector ring inserted into the magnet have been used in animal imagers and demonstrate potential for clinical systems. The reduced positron range created by the magnetic field also improves resolution.

PFI

Abbreviation of *Partial Flip* Imaging.

PGSE

Abbreviation for *Pulsed Gradient Spin Echo*.

pH measurement

The use of MR techniques to measure cellular pH, which may be important in cancer studies. The pH is a scale that reflects how acidic or alkaline something is, and is related to hydronium ion (H^+) concentration (pH is an abbreviation from pondus hydrogenii).

In MRS the chemical shift of phosphorus metabolites can be used to determine pH. Novel gadolinium-based contrast agents which are pH sensitive are also being developed.

See also *inorganic phosphate*.

Phantom

Any material or *test object*, which is designed to mimic the patient being imaged. The simplest designs consist of water filled spheres doped with a paramagnetic salt to reduce relaxation times to those seen in vivo (see *doping*). At high fields water must be replaced by oil to reduce the *standing wave artifact*. More complicated phantom designs consist of an arrangement of *perspex* or glass objects for comprehensive *quality assurance* tests.

Other more tissue equivalent materials may be used for instance *agarose gel* or *gelatine* (Fig. 66) (see *gel phantoms*).

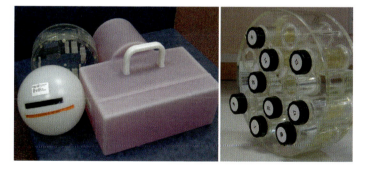

FIGURE 66 Types of *phantom* used in MRI quality assurance. (*Left*) A 1.5 T head sphere, a spatial resolution tool (Eurospin TO4) and a pink-colored oil phantom for 3.0 T. Liney G. MRI in clinical practice. London: Springer; 2006, p. 54. (*Right*) Gel phantoms providing a range of relaxation time values

References

Madsen EL, Fullerton GD. Prospective tissue-mimicking materials for use in NMR imaging phantoms. Magn Reson Imaging. 1982;1:135–141

Pharmacokinetic modeling

Computationally intensive method of applying a real physiological model to *dynamic contrast enhancement* data to determine tissue-specific parameters or descriptors. Common quantitative measures include the permeability constant (K^{TRANS}) which is often displayed in the form of a *parameter map* (Fig. 67).

See also *GKM*.

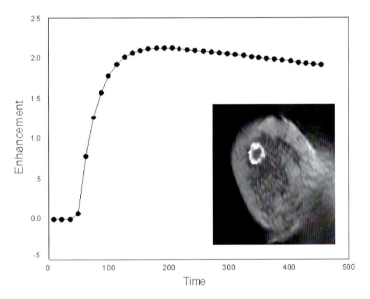

FIGURE 67 Example of *pharmacokinetic modeling* of breast tumor uptake during a chemotherapy trial. The plot shows the enhancement curve obtained from the tumor which has been fitted to a two compartment model. When this is done a pixel-by-pixel basis a parameter map of the transfer constant (K^{TRANS}) can be obtained (*inset*) which displays high peripheral enhancement

References

Tofts PS. Modelling tracer kinetics in dynamic Gd-DTPA MR imaging, J Magn Reson Imaging. 1997;7:91–101

Phase

1. The description of the position on the "clock face" attributed to spins as they precess in the transverse plane. Initially, all the spins tipped into the transverse plane by the excitation pulse are said to be in phase. Subsequently, the frequency of each spin changes so that they have different positions or phases relative to each other (see *dephasing*).
2. Phase is also used in *dynamic* imaging to indicate the temporal position in a time course.

Phase correction

Manual or automated method of adjusting the phase of MRS data so that the peaks in the *spectrum* all point above the *baseline*. Phase correction may be zero order (involving a linear offset of phase) or first (or higher) order requiring a more complicated transformation.

Phase contrast

Technique used in MR angiography (see *MRA*) where the amount of phase change induced by flow along a gradient direction is used to provide the image contrast (Fig. 68).

See also *velocity encoding* and *even echo re-phasing*.

Phase encoding

The use of incremental applications of a gradient in order to spatially discriminate signal along a particular direction

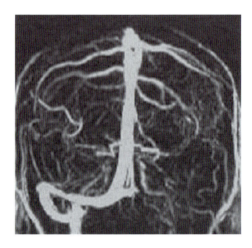

FIGURE 68 A *phase contrast* venogram of the sagittal and trans-verse sinus. Liney G. MRI in clinical practice. London: Springer; 2006, p. 111

by changes of *phase*. Unlike *frequency encoding* this process must be repeated hundreds of times; the number of increments of the phase-encoding gradient is equal to the image matrix in the phase encoding direction. This typically varies from 64 to 512 and governs the image *acquisition time*.

Signal aliasing can occur in this direction and is specifically called p*hase wrap*. Some other artifacts which are predominantly observed in the phase encoding direction are *ghosting*, *RF artifact* and *Gibbs artifact*.

Phase sensitive demodulator

Hardware component, which acts as a *double balanced mixer* in reverse i.e., it removes the RF component from the detected signal. This signal is then sent to the analog-to-digital converter (*ADC*) to be processed by the computer.

Phase (I, II, III…) trials

Referring to the different stages of testing associated with new MRI *contrast agents*, progressing from initial animal tests, through to small clinical trials and so forth, prior to their release onto the commercial market.

Phase wrap

Signal *aliasing* that specifically occurs in the phase encoding direction. In 3D imaging, phase wrap can also occur in the through-plane direction (Fig. 69).

See also *Moiré fringes*.

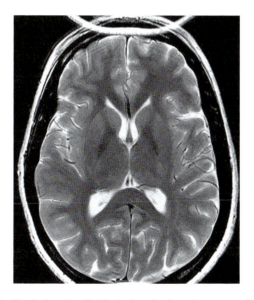

FIGURE 69 Reducing the field-of-view in the phase encoding direction has caused *phase wrap* with part of the anatomy being mismapped onto the top of the image. Liney G. MRI in clinical practice. London: Springer; 2006, p. 40

Phased array

See *array*.

Phi

Greek letter (φ) used to denote *phase*.

Philips

MRI vendor based in the Netherlands. Current products include whole-body 1.5 T (Intera & Achieva) and 3.0 T (Achieva) systems plus a 1.0 T *open scanner* (Panorama HFO).
www.healthcare.philips.com

PHIP

Abbreviation for *ParaHydrogen-Induced Polarization*.

Phosphocreatine

The main spectral resonance observed in phosphorous MRS, and used as the reference peak (see *PPM*). See Fig. 70.

Phosphodiesters

Spectral peak seen in phosphorous MRS at 3.0 ppm.

Phosphorus

The MR visible isotope of phosphorus is ^{31}P, and it is used in MRS for examining metabolism. It has a resonant frequency of 25.9 MHz at 1.5 T, and a chemical shift range of 30 ppm which means the spectral peaks are more easily distinguished compared to proton MRS. Phosphorus spectroscopy is also important in studies of cancer (e.g., hepatic tumors).

MR properties of ^{31}P:

Spin quantum number = 1/2
Sensitivity = 0.0663
Natural abundance = 100.00%
Gyromagnetic ratio = 17.23 MHz T^{-1}
See also *dual tune* (Fig. 70).

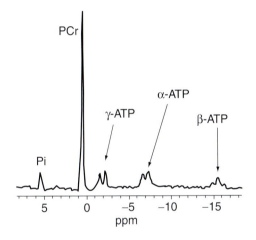

FIGURE 70 A single voxel *phosphorus* spectrum acquired from a healthy calf muscle in a study of metabolism. Note the wide dispersion and excellent SNR compared to proton (see Fig. 53). The peaks are *Pi* inorganic phosphate; *PCr* phosphocreatine and the three peaks from adenosinetriphosphate

Photoplethysmograph

A light transducer used for monitoring the patient's pulse from either their fingers or toes in *peripheral pulse gating*. Changes in blood volume in the nail bed alter the light reflected back to the photodetector.

PI

Abbreviation for *parallel imaging*.

Pianissimo

Name of the Toshiba technology for their *vacuum bore* design to reduce *acoustic noise* from the gradients (literally meaning "go quietly").

Picker

Former MRI vendor that changed its name to Marconi in 1999 and was later bought by Philips in 2001. Some old systems and terminology are still in current use.

PILS

Acronym for Parallel Imaging with Localized Sensitivities. A *parallel imaging* technique that is similar to *SMASH*.

Pillar

Referring to a specific design of an *open scanner* consisting of a vertical field produced from two pole-pieces which are separated by either two or four pillars to provide access to the patient.

Pixel

The smallest part of the image and derived from the words "picture element." It is defined by the field-of-view divided by the matrix size. In practice each pixel has a finite slice thickness and is therefore more correctly termed a *voxel*.

The pixel value gives the signal intensity at that point in the image and in a *parameter map* it indicates the actual value of the parameter.

Planck's constant

See *h*.

pMRI

Shorthand for *positional MRI*.

PNR

Abbreviation of Peak-to-Noise Ratio. It is the spectroscopy equivalent value to the measure of *SNR* used in imaging. It is usually measured as either the *peak amplitude* or the *peak area* divided by the *baseline* signal in the spectrum.

PNS

Abbreviation for *Peripheral Nerve Stimulation*.

Point spread function

Abbreviated to PSF. A mathematical description of the response of the imaging system to a point in the object which is a function of the number of phase encoding steps used. It is the spatial analog of modulation transfer function (see *MTF*). In effect, the PSF describes two things: the proportion of signal from any given voxel which is displaced into other voxels and the true voxel width.

See also *voxel bleeding*.

POMP

Acronym for Phase Offset MultiPlanar. A GE sequence for *simultaneous excitation*.

Positional MRI

Imaging performed with the patient in a variety of physiologically relevant positions rather than lying in the horizontal position of a conventional scanner. Sometimes written as pMRI.

See also *Fonar* and *C-Scan*.

Positive enhancement integral

A measurement made from *dynamic contrast enhancement* data that is a summation of the total signal above the baseline.

See also *area under the curve*.

Posterior

Referring to the rear side of patient anatomy. For a conventional *supine position*, it is at the bottom of an axial image and the right of a sagittal image (see Figs. 3 and 82).

See also *anterior*.

ppm

Abbreviation for Parts Per Million. The common reference scale used to report metabolite peaks in MRS. Each nucleus has a standard reference peak, which is set to 0 ppm. Other peaks are then quoted in terms of the frequency difference from this reference:

$$\text{ppm} = 10^6 \times (\upsilon - \upsilon_{\text{REF}}) / \upsilon_{\text{REF}}$$

where υ, and $υ_{REF}$ are the frequencies of the metabolite and the reference peaks.

For ^{1}H and ^{13}C the reference is tetramethylsilane (*TMS*). This gives water its characteristic *chemical shift* of 4.77 ppm. In ^{31}P the reference is phosphocreatine.

The advantage of using the ppm scale is that it is independent of field strength.

See *also chemical shift*.

PQRST wave

The terminology used to describe the various features of a characteristic ECG (electrocardiograph) wave pattern. This comprises of an initial P wave which is associated with atrial contraction. There then follows the QRS complex from ventricular contraction (with R being the peak signal) followed by the T wave at ventricular rest. In some cases a U wave is also observed. Cardiac gated images are triggered from successive R to R peaks (the *RR interval*).

In *peripheral pulse gating* the peak signal appears approximately 250 ms after the R peak from an ECG.

Preamp

Part of the receiver system, which moderately amplifies the inherently weak MR signal with a minimal addition of noise.

See also *ADC* and *phase sensitive demodulator*.

Pre-emphasis

A method of compensating for the effects of *eddy currents* by using distorted current waveforms for the gradient coils. When these are used in conjunction with the eddy current effects the combined result is to produce the desired linear field.

Precession

The motion experienced by the nuclear magnetic *moment* under the influence of an external magnetic field. The spin angular momentum of the nucleus means that rather than simply align with the field it traces out a cone around the direction of the field. A commonly used analogy is the motion of a spinning top in the Earth's gravitational field. The frequency of this precession is given by the Larmor equation (see *Larmor frequency*).

Precessional frequency

Synonym for *Larmor frequency*.

Pregnancy

Currently it is advised that pregnant women within the first trimester should not be scanned unless absolutely necessary. Although there is no evidence to suggest there are any harmful effects, the fetus is potentially more sensitive to the effects of *RF heating* and *acoustic noise*. When scans do take place, *contrast agents* are avoided as they are known to cross the placenta (Fig. 71).

See also *contraindications*.

Prepared

Expression used to describe an imaging sequence that is preceded by some additional RF excitation, for example a fat saturation pulse or an inversion pulse.

Pre-scan

An automatic routine performed by the scanner prior to each imaging scan. It involves several steps such as

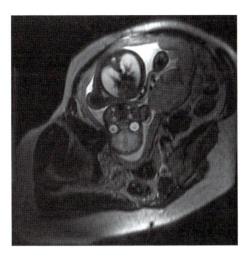

FIGURE 71 Image of the fetus in late *pregnancy*

shimming the prescribed volume (see *shim*) and tuning the RF coil to the *center frequency*. In addition the receiver and transmitter amplifiers are appropriately adjusted by playing out the sequence with zero phase encoding in order to produce the maximum signal amplitude. In some cases the pre-scan may fail to reach a certain tolerance and it can be manually optimized by the operator. For MRS, additional operations may also be included in the pre-scan e.g., *water suppression*.

PRESS

Acronym for Point RESolved Spin echo. A spectroscopy localisation sequence based on the signal from a spin echo. It uses a 90°–180°–180° pulse sequence in the presence of slice selection gradients in each orthogonal direction to excite a small *voxel*. The sequence has inherently better signal-to-noise than *STEAM* although minimum echo times are longer. PRESS also exhibits chemical-shift related mis-registration which can be improved by using larger bandwidths in techniques such as *PROSE*.

References

Bottomley PA. Spatial localization in NMR spectroscopy in vivo. Ann NY Acad Sci. 1987;508:333–348
    See also *TEA-PRESS*

PRESTO

Acronym, which stands for PRinciples of Echo Shifting with a Train of Observations. A sequence utilized by Philips as a whole-head fMRI or perfusion scan which is a *steady state* based EPI acquisition. The sequence is prone to motion artifacts.

References

Liu G, Sobering G, Duyn J, Moonen CTW. A functional MRI technique combining principles of echo-shifting with a train of observations (PRESTO). Magn Reson Med. 1993;30:764–768

Primary image

The gold standard data set to which the *secondary image* is fused or registered. It usually has the better resolution and volume coverage of the two image sets.
    See also *fusion* and *registration*.

Primovist

Commercial name of a *Liver-specific contrast agent* containing *gadolinium*. It has a generic name of gadoxetic acid disodium and a chemical name of Gd-EOB-DTPA.

PROBE

Acronym for PROton Brain Examination. GE's single or multi-voxel MRS sequence primarily used in the brain.

See also *PROSE*.

Profile phantom

A test object consisting of angled glass plates and used for measuring the nominal *slice profile*. A pixel intensity profile is taken along the plates which produces an inverted signal peak that is related to the slice thickness, b, by:

$$b = FWHM \times \tan \alpha$$

where *FWHM* is the full width at half maximum height of the inverted peak (in units of distance) and α is the angle of the plate.

Usually measurements are taken from plates of opposite angulation and a geometric mean is used which accounts for slight misalignment of the phantom (up to $5°$). A 10% tolerance is acceptable for slice thickness.

An alternative method utilizes an angled wedge in which case the pixel profile has to be first differentiated in order to obtain the slice profile (Fig. 72).

ProHance

Commercial name of a gadolinium based contrast agent from Bracco. It is similar to *Gd-DOTA* but one CO^- group is replaced with $CH(OH)(CH_3)$ resulting in a non-ionic complex. Its generic name is Gadoteridol.

Projectile

The result of a *ferromagnetic* object brought close to the scanner. Strong fields are induced within the object, which propel it into the scanner bore. The force of attraction is

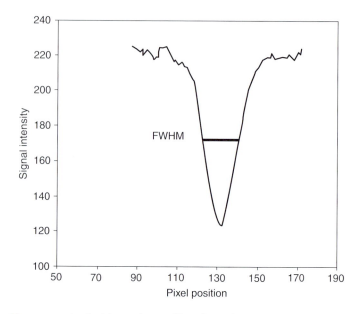

FIGURE 72 A pixel intensity profile taken along the angled plate in a *profile phantom.* The FWHM value used in the calculation of slice thickness is shown

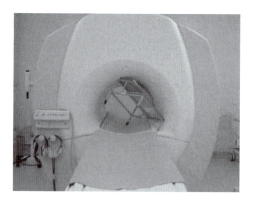

FIGURE 73 An illustration of the *projectile* effect. Liney G. MRI in clinical practice. London: Springer; 2006, p. 28

proportional to the mass of the object and inversely proportional to the square of its distance from the field.

Weakly ferromagnetic objects deemed safe at 1.5 T may not be safe at 3.0 T and a *deflection angle test* should be performed.

In the US, the FDA now support the use of a three-level classification system with appropriate labeling to indicate safety of devices (see *MR compatible*) (Fig. 73).

Projection fibers

Type of *white matter fibers* that connect the brain with the spinal cord.

Projection reconstruction

The original method of MR image reconstruction based on a series of projections acquired at many different angles.

See also *filtered back projection* and *Fourier transformation*.

Prone position

Imaging with the patient lying on their front for example in a conventional breast MR examination.

See also *supine position*.

PROPELLER

Acronym for Periodically Rotated Overlapping ParallEL Lines with Enhanced Reconstruction. A *radial k-space* sequence from GE. This reduces the effects of non-periodic motion and susceptibility artifacts. Other manufacturer equivalent techniques include BLADE (Siemens), RADAR (Hitachi), MULTIVANE (Philips) and JET (Toshiba) (Fig. 74).

See also *k-space trajectory*.

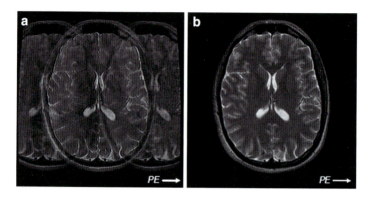

FIGURE 74 (*Left*) An image of a volunteer who was asked to deliberately move his head during the scan producing severe ghosting. (*Right*) The test is repeated with *PROPELLER* in order to remedy the motion artifacts. Copyright institute of physics and engineering in medicine 2008. Reproduced from 'Liney GP, Brackenbridge R, Dobbs M, K-space: the final frontier. SCOPE 2008;10–13. Institute of Physics and Engineering in Medicine 2008' with kind permission

PROSE

GE spectroscopy sequence specifically designed for use in the prostate (acronym of PROstate Spectroscopy Examination). It utilizes a *spectral-spatial pulse* in order to reduce misregistration and improve lipid suppression. The shape and narrow bandwidth of the excitation pulse is such that the lipid peak at 1.3 ppm is virtually absent (<1% signal), and only a small residual (5% signal) water peak is present which can be used as a chemical shift reference (see *PPM*).

PROSET

Philips utilization of a *binomial pulse* for fat suppression.

Proton

A sub-atomic particle of the nucleus that has a mass of 1.673×10^{-27} kg and a charge equal but opposite to that of an *electron*.

In the context of MRI the term "proton" usually refers to the spin of the common isotope of the hydrogen atom which consists of a single proton.

See also *hydrogen* and *deuterium*.

Proton decoupling

The action of a sequence designed to actively decouple proton resonances in order to improve the discrimination of other nuclei.

See also *nuclear overhauser effect*.

Proton density

Abbreviated to PD and sometimes given the Greek symbol rho (ρ). It is equal to the number of proton spins per unit volume of tissue. This is effectively equivalent to the amount of water (and fat) present. Proton density may differ from the true water content due to short T_2 components, which are not seen in MRI. Proton density (unlike T_1 and T_2) is not routinely quantified.

Proton density weighted

Image weighting where the T_1 and T_2 effects are minimized so that the contrast of the image is determined primarily by the spin (proton) density. This requires a short TE and long TR.

Proton-density weighted images may be used for pre-contrast T_1 correction in *dynamic contrast enhancement* data. They also demonstrate the white and gray matter differences in the brain. At long TR (12 s) CSF appears bright (100% PD), followed by gray matter (78%) and white matter (70%).

References

Gutteridge S, Ramanathan C, Bowtell R. Mapping the absolute value of M_0 using dipolar field effects. Magn Reson Med. 2002;47:871–879

Proximity limits

The maximum *fringe field* that specific objects can be safely placed in. Some typical values are listed below:

Inside 30 G: stainless steel, non-ferromagnetic objects
Outside 30 G: ECG monitors, unrestrained ferromagnetic objects
Outside 10 G: credit cards, floppy discs, X-ray tubes
Outside 5 G: pacemakers, public access etc
Outside 3 G: moving cars etc
Outside 1 G: TVs, monitors (CRT), CT & PET scanners
Outside 0.5 G: Railways, gamma cameras.

References

McAtamney P, Shaw D. Siting and installation. In: Practical NMR imaging. Foster MA, Hutchison JM, editors. Oxford: IRL Press; 1987

Pseudogating

Term used to describe the coincidental synchronicity between the signal acquisition and cardiac motion leading to clearly defined images which appear to have been gated.
    See also *gating*.

Pseudolayering

The banding appearance that can occur in the bladder due to variations in contrast agent concentration. Towards the base of the bladder where concentrations are high, the T_2 shortening effect of *gadolinium* agents predominates, resulting in a low signal intensity. Above this, at lower concentrations, a bright signal is observed due to normal T_1 relaxation effects.

See also *relaxivity*.

References

Elster AD, Sobel WT, Hinson WH. Pseudolayering of Gd-DTPA in the urinary bladder. Radiology. 1990;174:379

PSF

Abbreviation for *Point Spread Function*.

PSIF

A *steady state* sequence with the pulse diagram (and name) being the reverse of the *FISP* sequence. It has a prominent T_2 weighting.

Pu

Abbreviation for Pick-Up and used on Philips systems to denote the measurement of signal gain which is adjusted during the *pre-scan*.

Pulse

See *RF pulse*.

Pulse Controller

Hardware component, which manages the timing of the *spectrometer* and *gradients* during the imaging sequence.

Pulsed gradient spin echo

Abbreviated to PGSE. The generic name for the *Stejskal-Tanner* diffusion weighted imaging sequence.
  See also *DWI*.

Pulse programming

The creation and manipulation of a non-standard *pulse sequence* by the operator in order to implement user-specific imaging techniques. Typically involves thousands of lines of code.

Pulse sequence

A set of RF and gradient pulses of fixed duration and separation, which are used to produce an MR image. The sequence is usually represented in a *pulse sequence diagram*.

Pulse sequence diagram

Commonly used schematic representation of a *pulse sequence*. A separate line is used to display the action of the RF pulses, the gradients in each orthogonal direction and the signal that is generated. The gradients are shown as rectangles with the area representing the amplitude and duration, drawn either above or below the baseline to indicate a positive or negative sense.

Pulse train

A series of closely spaced RF pulses. Used for example in *steady state* or *burst imaging*.

PURE

The name for the GE method of improving RF coil uniformity that requires a calibration scan to be acquired.
See also *coil uniformity correction*.

P-value

Abbreviation for probability value. It is used to interpret the result of some statistical test. A result with a low P-value indicates a significant result (e.g., $P < 0.05$ is equivalent to only a 5% probability that the result has occurred by chance).
See also *t-test*, *bonferroni correction*, *correlation coefficient* and *statistical errors*.

References

Everitt BS. Medical statistics from A to Z. Cambridge: Cambridge University Press; 2003. ISBN: 0521532043

Q

Q

1. Used to denote the *imaginary* signal or channel of a *quadrature* RF coil.
2. A shorthand for *quality factor*.

Quadrature

The use of two *receiver* coils set 90° apart to detect the signal from two channels. Measuring the signal twice represents an improvement in SNR of √2 compared to non-quadrature (or *linearly polarized*) coils. The detected signal may be reconstructed from either component (termed *real* and *imaginary*) or from the phase of the signal. More typically the magnitude of the signal components is used. Errors involved in this quadrature detection lead to *ghosting*. Quadrature *transceiver* coils are also more efficient at transmitting RF power and therefore produce less *SAR* in the patient.

See also *RF coils*.

Quality factor

Also known as Q factor. This is a measure of the tuning characteristic of the RF coil and is defined by the amplitude and width of the resonant peak. A tall and narrow signal peak at resonance defines a high quality. RF coils are designed to work well for a range of Q factors since patient *loading* will alter this characteristic.

Quality assurance

The performance of routine quality control checks of the system or acceptance testing of a recently installed scanner. Usually, a daily quality assurance (QA) scan is acquired in a manufacturer specific *phantom* to visually establish scan quality. A more comprehensive but less frequent set of tests may be performed using specifically designed phantoms, and may include the following:

1. A homogenous or *floodfill phantom*, used for measuring *SNR*, *uniformity* and *ghosting*.
2. A phantom comprising an arrangement of plates for testing slice profile and *spatial resolution.*
3. A grid of known dimensions for estimating *geometric distortion.*
4. Test objects of different relaxation times to determine sequence contrast and relaxation time accuracy.

Usually tests are performed with the head and body coils using a standard spin-echo sequence. A more comprehensive QA program may include additional RF coils. Advanced sequences such as EPI, may be subject to additional testing such as measurement of *stability*.

Safety tests may also be performed and include the validation of the *fringe field* and a measurement of *acoustic noise* or temperature changes using specialist equipment (see *fluoroptic thermometer*).

Some systems offer a semi-automated QA protocol requiring minimal operator intervention.

See also *doping*, *profile phantom*, *resolution phantom* and *gel phantoms*.

References

Lerski R, De Wilde J, Boyce D, Ridgeway J. Quality control in magnetic resonance imaging, IPEM Report no. 80. York: IPEM; 1998

Quadscan

The name of a *simultaneous excitation* sequence from Toshiba.

Quadrupole-electric interactions

The mechanism, which dominates relaxation in nuclei with a spin *quantum number* greater or equal to 1 (e.g., ^{23}Na). These nuclei interact with the electric field of another nucleus rather than its magnetic field.

Quantum number

The discrete number used to describe the spin properties of a nucleus and usually denoted by the letter I.

It can take whole or half integer values for nuclei with an odd number of protons or neutrons. Most commonly studied nuclei have I = 1/2, and examples include ^{1}H, ^{31}P, ^{13}C and ^{19}F.

Nuclei with I greater than 1 exhibit *quadrupole-electric interactions*.

Nuclei with an even number of protons and neutrons have zero spin (I = 0), and are not *MR visible*. Examples include ^{16}O and ^{12}C.

The quantum number governs the possible number of energy states (or Zeeman levels) that are created in an external magnetic field, equal to 2I + 1. For the proton, with I = 1/2, there are two such states referred to as *spin up* and *spin down*.

An analogous quantum number (denoted m) is related to the longitudinal component of spin angular momentum and this can take a total of (2I+1) integer values from +I to –I.

Quench

The process, which occurs when a *superconducting magnet* loses its superconductivity and the *cryogens* begin to violently boil and escape out of the *cryostat*. The onset of a quench is indicated by a loud noise, tilting of the image and, unless the gases are properly vented, a white vapor emerging into the scan room, which causes an increase in pressure and drop in temperature. A quench may be described by the color of this vapor (normally "white" or more seriously "black," which indicates the permanent loss of the magnet). In the event of a quench, the gas should leave through a quench pipe which emerges from the top of the scanner and into the ceiling. On some older systems this can be seen separately from the *cold head* (see Fig. 48).

Failure to vent the gas may result in risk of asphyxia or frostbite for the patient and an oxygen monitor is used in the scan room to provide an appropriate warning.

See also *boil-off*.

QUEST

Acronym for the sequence called QUick Echo-Split imaging Technique. A type of *burst imaging* sequence using irregularly spaced RF pulses.

Quiet

The name for a type of gradient coil that uses *acoustic damping* to reduce *acoustic noise*.

QUICK 3D

A dynamic 3D volume sequence from Toshiba. Equivalent to *THRIVE*.

QUIPSS

Type of *arterial spin labeling* sequence employing saturation as opposed to inversion as the labeling method. It is an acronym of QUantitative Imaging of Perfusion using a Single Subtraction.

R

R

Used to denote the *real* signal or channel of a *quadrature* RF coil.

R_1

1. Commonly used shorthand for the longitudinal relaxation rate $(=1/T_1)$ with units of s^{-1}.
2. R1 (no lowercase number) is used on GE systems to denote the gain of the first *receiver*.

R_2

1. The transverse relaxation rate $(=1/T_2)$ with units of s^{-1} and normally written with the number in lowercase. Its measurement has been shown to correlate with hepatic iron content in patients with "iron-overload."
2. R2 (no lowercase number) is used on GE systems to denote the gain of the second *receiver*.

R_2^*

The effective transverse relaxation rate $(=1/T_{2*})$ with units of s^{-1}. Pronounced "R2 star," it is the analog of T_2^*. Measurements of this value have been used in cancer studies to probe tumor *hypoxia*. Long values of R_2^* imply poor oxygenation and therefore increased radioresistance (Fig. 75).

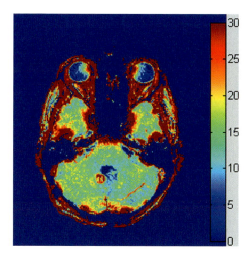

FIGURE 75 A map of R_2* demonstrates a hypoxic tumor (scale is in units of s^{-1})

RA

Abbreviation for *Relative Anisotropy*.

RADAR

An acronym for RADial Acquisition Regime. Hitachi's version of motion correction using a *radial k-space* acquisition.
    See also *k-space trajectory*.

Radial k-space

Referring to a variety of techniques that acquire *k-space* in a radial manner to provide a sequence that is robust with respect to motion. The method involves traversing k-space at a number of different angles (or "blades") with the center being oversampled. Undersampling of the radial trajectories can cause radial streaks in the background of the recon-structed image. Vendor specific implementations include *PROPELLER* (GE), *BLADE* (Siemens), *RADAR* (Hitachi), *MULTIVANE* (Philips) and *JET* (Toshiba).

See also *k-space trajectory*.

Radiotherapy

The use of radioactive sources or external high energy beams to treat tumors whilst sparing normal tissue. The treatment dose is given over a series of fractions.

See also *brachytherapy* and *Linac*.

Radiotherapy planning

The use of MRI to provide soft-tissue detail to improve the delineation of treatment volumes. Conventional CT images, used for electron density calculations, are registered with MRI. Spatial inaccuracies due to *geometric distortion* must be minimized or accounted for. In certain situations where the anatomy is homogenous, e.g., in the brain, an overall assumed electron density can be used and only MRI is needed for planning. For optimum registration with CT, the MRI exami-nation should be acquired in the same treatment position. This usually involves a temporary flat table top and some fixation device (e.g., restraining mask). Dedicated flexible RF coils that accommodate this set-up can be used to provide optimum imaging (Fig. 76).

References

Beavis AW, Gibbs P, Dealey RA, Whitton VJ. Radiotherapy treat-ment planning of brain tumours using MR images alone. Br J Radiol. 1998;71:544–548

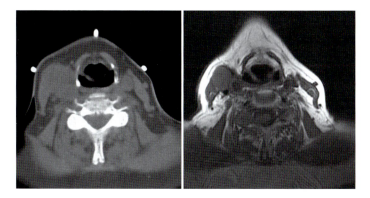

FIGURE 76 (*Left*) A CT image of a head-and-neck tumor and a corresponding (*right*) MRI used to provide extra soft-tissue delineation for *radiotherapy planning*

RACE

Acronym for Real-time ACquisition and velocity Evaluation. A 1D technique where a very rapid sequence is used to acquire data across a vessel and measure the velocity of blood.

RADIANCE

Name of a dynamic 3D volume sequence for breast imaging from Toshiba that is equivalent to *VIBRANT*.

Radians

An alternative unit for describing *flip* angles. 2π radians is equal to 360° (a 90° pulse is therefore referred to as $\pi/2$). Note that *angular frequency* is measured in radians per second and is given by $2\pi f$ where f is the frequency in Hertz.

RAM-FAST

Acronym for Rapid Acquisition Matrix *FAST*.

Ramp up/down

The process by which the magnetic (B_0) field is turned on or off in a scanner. In a *superconducting magnet* an external power supply is applied and then a superconducting switch is used to short-circuit the magnet once the desired field is established. Ramp time may also be used to describe gradients reaching maximum amplitude although the term *rise time* is more accurate.

Ramp sampling

The technique of sampling the MRI signal while the gradient is yet to achieve its maximum amplitude i.e., during the *rise time* of the gradient. This improves the efficiency of the image acquisition.

Ramped RF pulses

RF excitation pulses with variable flip angles in a time-of-flight sequence (see *TOF*). The flip angle is increased along the slice direction to combat the saturation of the flowing signal and maintain the in-flow enhancement effect.

See also *TONE*.

RAPID

Name of the image-based *parallel imaging* acquisition utilized on Hitachi systems.

RARE

Acronym for Rapid Acquisition with Relaxation Enhancement. The original name for generic sequences such as *FSE*, *TSE* and *FAISE*.

References

Hennig J, Nauerth A, Freidburg H. RARE imaging: A fast imaging method for clinical MR. Magn Resn Med. 1986;3:823–833

Raw data

The acquired MRI or MRS data prior to any manipulation. Specifically the term should be reserved for the time domain data acquired prior to *Fourier transformation*. It may also be used to refer to an image before post-processing in order to obtain some *parameter map* (also known as source data).

Raysum

A method of visualizing image data in 3D. A set of mathematical paths are traversed through the original image data and the signal intensity values are summed at each point to create the final projection. This is in contrast to a *maximum intensity projection* which utilizes the highest signal value along each path.

RC

DICOM annotation for Respiratory Compensation.

Readout gradient

An old and less commonly used term for the *frequency encoding* gradient.

Real

Signal from one of the receiver channels in *quadrature* detection. Usually abbreviated to the letter R.

See also *imaginary*.

Real time fMRI

An *fMRI* acquisition, where images are acquired and activation maps are processed "on the fly" so that the study can be continually monitored to determine the compliance of the patient or terminate the acquisition (e.g., GE's BrainWave).

Receiver

An *RF coil* and the associated hardware used to detect the MR signal. During the *pre-scan*, the receiver and *transmitter* are adjusted to accommodate the range of signal. GE systems use R1 and R2 values to report the receiver gains. Similarly there are two FFT scales for Siemens scanners. Philips systems report a pick-up coil (Pu) and noise (Ns) measurement.

See also *bandwidth*, *quadrature* and *optical RF*.

Reconstruction

The process of *Fourier transformation* and display of the image or spectrum following data acquisition. For most image techniques this is done with near simultaneity so that there is no appreciable delay, although large dynamic volumes and some fat-water only imaging techniques can take longer. Reconstruction speeds are quoted in seconds per 256×256 image and may be 0.01 s or better.

Errors in the reconstruction process lead to a characteristic *herringbone artifact*.

Rectangular FOV

A non-square imaging field-of-view (FOV) obtained by reducing the dimension in the phase encoding direction with a concomitant reduction in the matrix size. This is useful for avoiding phase wrap or imaging rectangular shaped anatomy in shorter scan times. It may be denoted as RFOV together with a percentage value to indicate the fraction of the reduction.

Reduced flip angle

A smaller than normal *flip angle* used in sequences with long echo trains in an attempt to reduce the total *SAR* given to the patient. For example a 150° refocusing pulse may be used instead of the normal 180° in a fast spin-echo (*FSE*) sequence. Note that *partial flip* angle is more commonly used to refer to reduced excitation pulses.

Refocusing pulse

A specific application of an RF pulse which is used to recover the phase of spins. If it is applied at time TE/2 after an initial RF pulse it will produce a *spin echo* at time TE. The optimum refocusing occurs when the refocusing *flip angle* is 180° (or π *radians*) (Fig. 77).

Reformat

The display of image data in a different plane from the one in which it was acquired e.g., the data may be acquired axially, but subsequently reformatted in the coronal plane. Reformatting may also be performed in an oblique orientation. For best results the images should be acquire in thin contiguous slices or from 3D sequences. Also denoted MPR or multi-planar reformat.

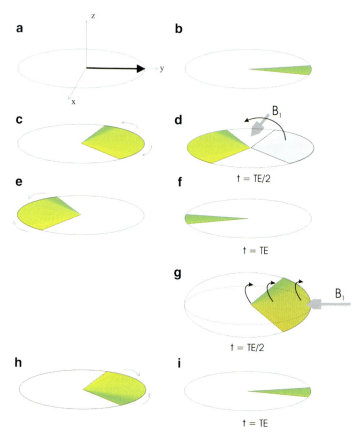

FIGURE 77 Diagram showing the action of a *refocusing pulse* in the production of a spin-echo. (**a–c**) The spins dephase in the transverse plane so the faster spins (*yellow*) are ahead of the slower spins (*green*). At time TE/2 the refocusing pulse is applied in either the x-direction (**d**) or y-direction (**g**). In either case the phase of the spins is reversed so an equal time later the faster spins catch-up and form a spin-echo (**h, i**). Liney G. MRI in clinical practice. London: Springer; 2006, p. 6

Registration

Term relating to the alignment of two image data sets which are generally (but not always) from the same examination. Examples include matching a set of dynamic contrast enhanced images to correct for patient movement between successive time points (e.g., *BRACE*). Registration can be classified as rigid or non-rigid body. Rigid-body registration correct for rotations and translations only whereas non-rigid body registration permits changes in shape. Sometimes referred to as image *fusion*.

Region-of-interest

More commonly seen as the abbreviation *ROI*.

Relative anisotropy

Often abbreviated to RA. Anisotropy index obtained from diffusion tensor imaging (*DTI*). It is given by:

$$RA = \sqrt{\frac{\left((\lambda_1 - \lambda_2)^2 + (\lambda_2 - \lambda_3)^2 + (\lambda_3 - \lambda_1)^2 \right)}{\lambda_1 + \lambda_2 + \lambda_3}}$$

where $\lambda_1 \ldots \lambda_3$ are the *eigenvalues* from the diffusion tensor. The denominator of the equation is equal to the *trace*. A more commonly used parameter is *fractional anisotropy*.

Relaxation

The mechanisms which effect excited spins once the RF energy (B_1 pulse) has been removed, leading to a return to the equilibrium position where the net magnetization is aligned with the main magnetic field. The spins lose phase coherence due to transverse relaxation and then signal recovers along the z-direction due to longitudinal relaxation (Fig. 78).

See also T_1, T_2 and T_2^*.

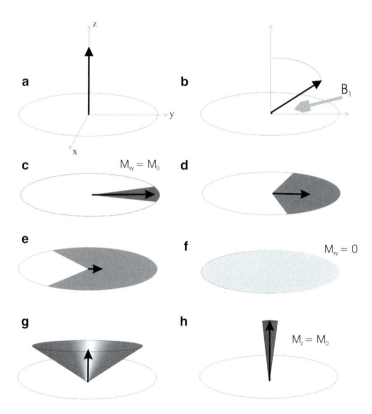

FIGURE 78 Diagram showing the mechanism of *relaxation*. (**a**) The net magnetization is initially aligned with B_0. (**b**) A B_1 pulse is applied which tips the magnetization into the transverse plane. (**c–f**) The transverse component decays to zero due to T_2 relaxation. (**g, h**) The longitudinal component regrows in the direction of B_0 due to T_1 relaxation. Liney G. MRI in clinical practice. London: Springer; 2006, p. 4

Relaxivity

The property of *contrast agents*, which determines their ability to shorten relaxation times. Changes in relaxation time are given by:

$$R_1^{'} = R_1 + k_1 \times D$$
$$R_2^{'} = R_2 + k_2 \times D$$

where D is the concentration of the contrast agent, R_1 (or R_2) is the native tissue relaxation rate, R_1' (R_2') is the new rate and k_1 (k_2) is the contrast agent relaxivity.

Gadolinium based agents have similar values for both k_1 and k_2. The values for *Gd-DTPA* at 1.5 T are 4.5 and 5.5 $mM^{-1}s^{-1}$ respectively. However, T_1 relaxation is the dominant effect as in vivo T_1 values are inherently longer than T_2.

SPIO agents have much greater relaxivity values with $k_2 \gg k_1$ (e.g., 165 and 25 $mM^{-1}s^{-1}$). This means that these agents produce a greater T_2 relaxation effect.

See also *doping*.

Relief artifact

See *chemical shift artifact ("of the second kind")*.

Repetition time

See *TR*.

RES agents

Abbreviation for *ReticuloEndothelial System agents*.

Research mode

An unrestricted operational level of the scanner, usually requiring ethics permission, where patient exposure should be monitored in case of unwanted side effects.

See also *bio-effects*, *normal mode*, *controlled mode* and *safety limits*.

Residual water

The left-over water peak observed in ^{1}H MRS following the application of *water suppression*. The water signal is typically reduced by a factor of several hundred times, but the remaining signal may be still be sufficient to be used as a chemical shift reference (see *ppm*).

Resistive magnet

A type of scanner utilizing an electromagnet, which can be turned on or off, and requiring large amounts of electrical power (50–100 kW) and usually water-cooling. A resistive magnet produces a lower field strength than a *superconducting magnet*. They can be air-cored or iron-cored, providing fields of up to 0.2 and 0.6 T respectively. Resistive windings can also be used to augment the field produced by a *permanent magnet* in some hybrid designs, reducing the overall power and weight of the individual types.

Resolution phantom

A test object comprising of a series of glass or *perspex* plates with varying separations and thickness (bar patterns) for evaluating spatial resolution. A visual inspection of a pixel profile taken across these plates indicates whether the appropriate resolution has been achieved. A threshold of 50%

modulation (the relative peaks and troughs) is acceptable. Both phase and frequency should be tested, by swapping encoding directions and changing the phantom orientation. Usually the resolution is poorer in the phase encoding direction. An alternative approach is determining the modulation transfer function (see *MTF*) from an angled block (Fig. 79).

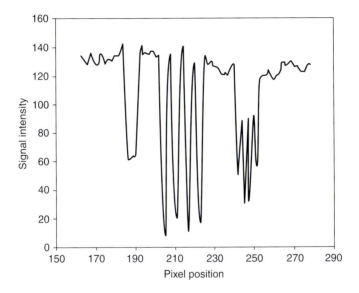

FIGURE 79 A pixel intensity profile taken across a set of bar patterns (0.5, 2.0 and 1.0 mm) in the *resolution phantom*, (shown in Fig. 66), in order to demonstrate the spatial resolution of an image sequence. Liney G. MRI in clinical practice. London: Springer; 2006, p. 58

Resonant frequency

See *Larmor frequency*.

Resonant offset artifacts

See *banding artifacts*.

Resovist

Commercial name for a *USPIO* type contrast agent for liver imaging. It has been developed by Bayer Schering Pharma AG and is more generally referred to as Ferrixan or Ferucarbotran, a *dextran*-coated iron oxide.

See also *liver-specific contrast agents*.

Respiratory compensation

Accommodating the motion caused by respiration by either employing some form of *respiratory gating* or utilizing short *breath hold* scans.

Respiratory gating

Synchronizing the imaging sequence to the periodicity of respiration in order to reduce motion artifacts. Previously this has required the use of pressure bellows or a belt placed around the patient to trace the breathing pattern and gate the images according to this measurement. Modern solutions include reduced scan times (see *breath hold*) or using a *navigator echo*.

REST

Abbreviation for REgional SaTuration. The name used by Philips to describe the saturation bands positioned outside the imaging volume to reduce flow and motion artifacts. The *moving saturation pulse* version is known as Travel REST.

RESTORE

Name given to Siemens' *driven equilibrium* sequence.

Restricted diffusion

The process of *diffusion* which has been limited by cell boundaries. It may be investigated by acquiring diffusion-weighted
images at several values of the *diffusion time*. In free diffusion,
the mean displacement is proportional to the diffusion time.
However if there is restriction the measured diffusion (see
ADC) will reach a plateau as diffusion time is increased.
    See also *DWI*.

References

Le Bihan D. Molecular diffusion, tissue microdynamics and micro-
structure. NMR Biomed. 1995;8:375–386

Reticuloendothelial system agents

Also abbreviated to RES agents. A particular type of contrast
agent taken-up by the Kupffer cells in the normal liver.
    See also *liver-specific contrast agents*.

REVEAL

The name for Siemens' whole body diffusion imaging
application.
    See also *DWIBS*.

Rewinding gradients

The use of gradients to re-phase spins at the end of a sequence
for example in *FSE* and *FISP* type sequences.

Reynolds number

A dimensionless quantity, which predicts the onset of turbulent flow (see *flow phenomena*). It is defined as the product

of fluid density, vessel diameter and velocity divided by viscosity. Generally laminar flow is present for Reynolds numbers less than 2,100.

RF

Shorthand for the Radio-Frequency component of the electromagnetic spectrum i.e., in the frequency range of 0 to 3,000 GHz, which includes radio waves, UHF, television and microwave. At 1.5 T the *Larmor frequency* of proton is 63.8 MHz which is at the lower end of the radio-frequency range.

RF antenna

Synonym for *RF coil*.

RF artifact

A distinctive striped line running along the phase encoding direction (i.e., perpendicular to the frequency direction) and caused by RF interference. The position and width of the artifact identifies the frequency and bandwidth of the likely source. Its characteristic appearance gives it the alternative name of zip (or zipper) artifact (Fig. 80).

See also *Faraday cage* and *FID artifact*.

RF burns

A skin burn to the patient caused by excessive *RF heating* in combination with a number of other contributory factors. These include direct contact with RF coils, skin-to-skin contact and use of high *SAR* scans. Devices and implants may also provide an increased risk. Care has to be taken with leads from external patient monitoring equipment. First, second

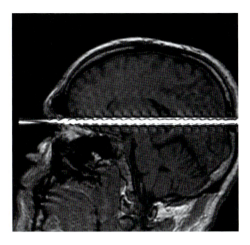

FIGURE 80   An extreme *RF artifact* seen in this image. The frequency encoding direction is top to bottom

and third degree burns have all been reported although this is extremely rare and virtually unknown below fields of 1.0 T.

References

Dempsey MF, Condon B, Hadley DM. Investigation of the factors responsible for burns during MRI. J Magn Reson Imaging. 2001;13:627–631

RF cage

See *Faraday cage*.

RF coil

The device placed on or around the anatomy of interest prior to imaging. This acts as a radio-frequency antenna that is tuned to the *Larmor frequency* and produces the B_1 magnetic field. This coil is known as the *transmitter*. A coil is also required to detect the signal, known as the *receiver*. Some coils act as a combined *transceiver*. Common types of RF coil include *surface coil*, *solenoid coil*, *birdcage coil* and *saddle coil*.

The resonant frequency ω of the coil is related to both its inductance, L and its capacitance C by:

$$\omega = \frac{1}{\sqrt{LC}}$$

The RF coil should be of similar size to the anatomy of interest to maintain good signal-to-noise ratio (*SNR*). This is to maximize signal from the imaged slice whilst minimizing the noise which comes from the entire *sensitive volume* of the coil (Fig. 81).

See also *head coil*, *body coil* and *wavelength*.

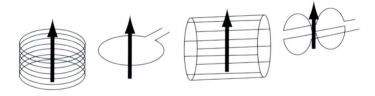

FIGURE 81 Diagram of various *RF coil* designs. (*Left to right*) A multiple turn solenoid, single turn surface coil, birdcage coil and saddle coil. All produce the B_1 field in the direction shown with the last three being most suited to conventional horizontal field systems while the solenoid is used in vertical fields

RF effects

The RF heating that occurs in tissue due to application of repetitive RF pulses (see *SAR*). This may be of particular concern in patients with thermoregulatory problems and in heat sensitive organs like the testis or in the fetus. Heating in implants or devices is of greater concern (see *RF burns*).

RF heating

The RF energy that is transmitted as part of the imaging process is converted to heat in the patient due to resistive losses and causes a potential safety risk (see *RF effects*). The amount of energy deposited in the patient is quantified by the specific absorption rate (*SAR*). This depends on a number of factors including field strength and RF pulse duration but it is also dependent on coil type and orientation.

Generally, there is a poor correlation between SAR and temperature rises. Temperature can be measured during a scan using an MR compatible *fluoroptic thermometer*. Many studies have demonstrated significant skin temperature rises of several degrees following continued RF exposure over long periods. Core temperature (measured sublingually) may also exhibit a slight increase but none of these changes are physiologically serious. The Adair model demonstrates that a core temperature rise of only 1°C occurs during 1 h exposure to 4 W kg^{-1} although this is dependent on ambient temperature. The distribution of temperature may not be uniform especially at higher field strengths where it is more likely to occur at the edges of a patient.

References

Adair ER, Berglund LG. On the thermoregulatory consequences of NMR imaging. Magn Reson Imaging. 1986;4:321–333

RF penetration

See *skin depth*.

RF power

The amount of RF energy required during the imaging sequence (and therefore deposited to the patient). The RF power (P) at a frequency ω_0 is given by:

$$P = 2\omega_0 B_1^2 V_c / \mu_0 Q$$

where V_c is the volume of the *RF coil* and Q is the *quality factor* of the coil. The value of Q drops with increasing frequency so that P is actually proportional ω_0^2. This necessitates the use of increased RF power at higher fields.

See also *SAR*.

RF pulse

The transient application of the magnetic component of an RF wave (referred to as the B_1 field) for the purposes of perturbing the net magnetization. The pulse must be applied at the *Larmor frequency* and also in a direction that is perpendicular to B_0. It is usually employed as an *excitation pulse* or a *re-focussing pulse*. The pulse can be described as being selective (a soft pulse) i.e., in the presence of a gradient field to influence only a finite section of spins, or non-selective (hard pulse) which affects the entire volume. The *pulse controller* unit, ensures the accurate timing and amplitude of the RF pulses.

See also *slice selection*.

RF shielding

Alternatively known as RF screening. This refers to the provision of a *Faraday cage* in the construction of the scan room. This is to eliminate radio-frequency interference which would otherwise cause an *RF artifact*. The cables and connections to the RF coils also need to be carefully shielded.

RF shimming

The optimisation of the B_1 field prior to imaging. This is essential at very high fields (>3.0 T) where poor RF penetration becomes problematic.

See also *skin depth*.

RF spoiling

See *Spoiling*.

RFA

Abbreviation for *Reduced flip angle*.

RFOV

See *Rectangular FOV*.

RG

DICOM annotation for Respiratory Gating.

Rho

Greek symbol (ρ) used to denote *proton-density*.

Rim enhancement

Characteristic appearance of the well-perfused periphery of a tumor, which preferentially enhances during a *contrast-enhanced* scan, while the necrotic center takes up little contrast. Also referred to as peripheral or centripetal enhancement. An example of this is shown in Fig. 67.

Ringing

A particular type of artifact seen at high-contrast interfaces (see *Gibb's artifact*). Also known as *truncation artifact*.

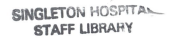

RISE

Acronym for Rapid Imaging Spin-Echo, a sequence similar to *FSE*.

Rise time

The finite time taken to achieve the maximum amplitude of the *gradient*. Typical rise times are several hundred μs. Also less commonly referred to as the *attack* of the gradient.

See also *fall time*.

ROAST

Acronym for Resonant Offset Averaging STeady state. A technique utilizing phase-cycled RF pulses to reduce *banding artifacts* in *True FISP* sequences

ROC curve

Abbreviation for Receiver Operating Characteristic curve. It is a plot of the sensitivity against 1-specificity for a particular diagnostic technique. It is a comparison of two operating characteristics at varying criteria and is also equivalent to a plot of the true positive rate against the false positive rate. A common way of reporting the information is using the *area under the curve* with higher values indicating a more accurate technique. Often used to chose between different imaging modalities e.g., MRI and ultrasound.

RODEO

Acronym for ROtating Delivery of Excitation Off resonance. A gradient echo sequence using RF pulses centered on either fat or water to suppress signal from one or the other. Also known as PROSET on Philips.

ROI

Commonly used abbreviation for Region-Of-Interest. A user-defined area of an image from which the pixel intensity values are measured.

References

Liney GP, Gibbs P, Hayes C, Leach MO, Turnbull LW. Dynamic contrast-enhanced MRI in the differentiation of breast tumours: user defined versus semi-automated region-of-interest. J Magn Reson Imaging. 1999;10:945–949

Rolling baseline

A slowly varying *baseline* that is introduced into an MRS spectrum due to *phase correction*. It can be removed by fitting a *spline* in-between the peaks and subtracting the result.

ROPE

Acronym for Respiratory Ordered Phase Encoding. A method of *respiratory compensation* using pressure bellows to monitor respiratory motion and re-ordering the k-space acquisition so that consecutive lines of data are acquired at similar points of the cycle.

It cannot be used in *FSE* sequences where the phase encoding order is governed by the echo times.

Rotating frame

The frame of reference in which the observer is also rotating at the *Larmor frequency* so that the spin appears stationary. This is adopted instead of the *laboratory frame* of reference in order to simplify the description of MRI. For example, as seen in the rotating frame, the application of the *excitation pulse* simply tips the spins into the transverse plane rather than the spiral motion away from B_0 that is observed in the laboratory frame.

RR interval

The time between consecutive parts of the ECG waveform used in the timing of gated sequences (see *ECG gating*). Typically the resting heart rate is around 75 bpm with an RR interval of 800 ms. This may be reduced to 400 ms during periods of stress or exercise.

See also *PQRST wave* and *trigger window*.

S

Saddle coil

A particular type of *RF coil* design, which produces the B_1 field perpendicular to the long-axis of the coil (see Fig. 81).

See also *birdcage coil*.

Safety limits

In the UK the MHRA (Medicines and Healthcare products regulatory agency) has published guidelines summarizing the latest recommendations from the Health Protection Agency (HPA, formerly the National Radiation protection Board, NRPB), the International Electrotechnical Commission (IEC) and the International Commission on Non-ionizing Radiation Protection (ICNIRP). Safe operation is stratified into normal mode (no effects), controlled mode (mild transient effects) and research mode (unrestricted exposure requiring monitoring).

Below is a summary of the currently accepted guidance for each of the main three magnetic field interactions in terms of exposure limits for patients.

- Static field: NRPB states that fields of 2.5 T (head) and 4.0 T (trunk) should not be exceeded routinely and this is increased to 4.0 T generally in controlled use. The IEC/ICNIRP values are <2 and 2–4 T respectively. All organizations say that ethics approval is needed above 4.0 T.
- Gradient fields: NRPB limits are $20\,\mathrm{T\,s^{-1}}$ for periods longer than 120 μs and $(2.4\times10^{-3})/t\,\mathrm{Ts^{-1}}$ for shorter periods. If the patient is monitored this can increase to $(60\times10^{-3})/t\,\mathrm{Ts^{-1}}$ for less than 3 ms periods. IEC states normal operation should not exceed 80% of *PNS* threshold and this may be

increased to 100% in a controlled environment. Hearing protection should be worn when noise levels exceed an ear-weighting level of 99 db(A).

- RF field: NRPB limits whole-body *SAR* to 1 W kg⁻¹ for exposure greater than 30 min although there is considerable variation depending on body part and duration. IEC/ICNIRP sets whole-body limits to 2 W kg⁻¹ (normal) and 4 W kg⁻¹ (controlled). In addition whole-body temperature rises are restricted to 0.5°C (normal) and 1.0°C (controlled) by NRPB, IEC and ICNIRP. SAR limits are based on moderate environmental conditions and should be adjusted according to ambient temperature and humidity.

For the latest guidelines the references below should be consulted.

See also *occupational exposure* and *bio-effects*.

References

Shellock FG. Magnetic resonance procedures: health effects and safety. Boca Raton: CRC Press; 2000. ISBN: 0849308747

http://www.mhra.gov.uk/Publications/Safetyguidance/DeviceBulletins/CON2033018

http://www.icnirp.de/documents/MR2004.pdf

http://www.hpa.org.uk/radiation/

http://www.iec.ch/

Kanal E. et al ACR guidance document for safe MR practices: 2007. AJR Am J Roentgenol. 2007;188:1447–1474

SAGE

Acronym for Spectroscopy Acquisition GE. A post-processing package for MR spectroscopy used with GE systems.

Sagittal

The imaging plane, which divides the patient into right and left i.e., the *slice selection*, is in the x direction and the in-plane directions are head to foot (superior to inferior) and anterior-posterior (Fig. 82).

See also *coronal*, *axial*, *oblique* and *anterior*.

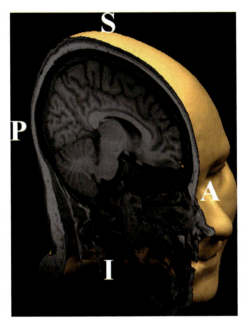

FIGURE 82 A 3D reconstruction of a brain volume which has been sliced in the *sagittal* plane. The image is labeled to indicate the anterior, posterior, superior and inferior directions

Saline

A small volume of saline (0.9% NaCl) is administered to the patient intravenously to ensure complete delivery of MR *contrast agents* (called a saline flush).

Saline may also be used to provide *loading* of the RF coil when imaging a test object.

Sampling rate

See *Nyquist frequency*.

SAR

Abbreviation for Specific Absorption Rate. It is the amount of RF power deposited as heat to the patient and is expressed in W kg^{-1}. This figure increases quadratically with field strength, necessitating the use of *reduced flip angle* sequences or *parallel imaging* techniques at 3.0 T. Current guidelines limit whole-body SARs to between 1 and 4 W kg^{-1} (see *safety limits*).

SAR is related to flip angle, α and *duty cycle, D* as follows:

$$SAR \propto B_0^2 \alpha^2 D$$

Studies have been performed to monitor the temperature rise in animals and also volunteers (see *RF heating*).

SAR also shows some dependence on *patient weight*, with a peak at around 60 kg and decrease thereafter.

SARGE

Acronym for Spoiled steady-state Acquisition Rewinded Gradient Echo. A *steady-state* sequence similar to *True FISP*. Hitachi use the abbreviation SG for SARGE and have sequences known as BASG (BAlanced SARGE), PBSG (Phase Balanced SARGE) and TRSG (Time Reversed SARGE).

Saturation bands

The graphical representation of the position and thickness of *saturation pulses*. An example of their use is shown in Fig. 58.

Saturation pulses

The utilization of slice selection in combination with dephasing gradients to remove signal, which may otherwise cause unwanted effects. For example, in flow compensation or outside MRS voxels.

See also *VSS*.

Saturation recovery

The use a 90° pulse and repeat acquisitions of signal at several different repetition times (TR) in order to measure the T_1 recovery. The signal is given by:

$$S \propto \left[1 - \exp(-TR/T_1)\right]$$

See also *inversion recovery*.

Saturated spins

The state of constant magnetization value (*partial saturation*) achieved at the end of the pulse sequence when $TR < T_1$.

Un-saturated spins have their full magnetization available at the end of the repetition time. This is either because $TR \gg T_1$ so the spins have fully relaxed or they have yet to be subjected to RF excitation in which case they are described as "fresh" spins, and is the basis of *in-flow enhancement*.

Scalar coupling

See *J-coupling*.

Scan assistant

An on-screen box that appears on a Siemens system to indicate the trade-off associated with changing certain imaging parameters.

Scan percentage

The figure used by Philips scanners to denote the reduction in k-space in a *partial k-space* acquisition.

Scan room

The specially constructed room that houses the MR scanner.
See also *Faraday cage* and *control room*.

Scan time

See *acquisition time*.

Scanning, 4D

A term often used to describe the acquisition of multiple 3D volumes with the fourth dimension referring to time e.g., in a dynamic contrast-enhanced *MRA*.
See also *time-resolved MRA*.

Scanogram

See *localiser*.

SCIC

GE acronym meaning Surface Coil Intensity Correction. A post-processing method used to improve the homogeneity of *surface coil* images.
See also *coil uniformity correction*.

Scout images

See *localiser*.

Screening

1. The action of going through a check-list of questions with the patient to ensure there are no contraindications for MRI (see *screening form*). The patient may require an *orbit X-ray* prior to examination if there are any concerns regarding previous shrapnel injuries.
2. Referring to an MRI examination that is used to check for an undiagnosed pathology (e.g., breast screening or *whole-body screening*).
3. The use of the *Faraday cage* to prevent RF interference may be termed RF screening but is more commonly known as *RF shielding.*

Screening constant

Alternative name for the *shielding constant.*

Screening form

The check-list that a radiographer goes through with the patient prior to their scan to ensure that there are no contraindications (this process is called screening). A typical form will consist of a series of safety queries regarding pregnancy status, adverse reactions to contrast agents, history regarding shrapnel injuries etc and identify any metallic objects which should be removed prior to entering the scan room.

Screenshot

An image produced from the capture of an on-screen graphical display rather than from real data. It will usually be saved in a graphics format (e.g., bitmap, tif etc.) rather than true *DICOM.*

SDNR

Abbreviation for Signal Difference to Noise Ratio. See *contrast-to-noise ratio*.

SE

Abbreviation for *spin echo*.

Secondary image

The dataset that is fused to the *primary image*. It usually has a reduced spatial resolution and smaller volume coverage compared to the primary image.

See also *fusion* and *registration*.

Seed point

A user-defined pixel, which forms the starting point for subsequent image processing, e.g., region growing, thresholding, fiber tracking etc.

Segmentation

The separation of connected pixels which are within a given signal intensity *threshold*. It permits the identification and measurement of tissue structures. An example of tissue segmentation is shown in Fig. 55.

Segmented k-space

A cardiac imaging technique, which permits multiple phases of the cardiac cycle to be imaged during a single breath-hold.

A small portion (called a segment) of k-space is filled for each frame in the cardiac cycle within each *RR interval*. For example, if there are 32 segments for a 128 matrix, this means 32 RR intervals (heartbeats) are required, each acquiring four lines of k-space (referred to as four views per segment). The number of possible frames is dependent on heart rate, the number of segments and repetition time (*TR*).

See also *cardiac MRI*.

SENSE

Acronym for SENSitivity Encoding. A *parallel imaging* method, similar to SMASH except it operates in the imaging domain. Images with a reduced number of phase encoding steps are unwrapped using knowledge of separate coil sensitivity profiles. It is commercially implemented by Philips. Siemens version is called mSENSE (or modified SENSE).

References

Pruessman KP, Weiger M, Scheidegger M, Boesiger P. SENSE: sensitivity encoding for fast MRI. Magn Reson Med. 1999;42:952–962

Sensitive volume

The volume of tissue from which the RF coil is able to detect signal and noise. This means it is prudent to select the smallest sized coil appropriate to the anatomy in order to optimize signal-to-noise ratio (*SNR)*.

Sequential

The acquisition of slices (or phases) in continuous order. This is the opposite of an *interleaved* acquisition.

Sequential k-space filling

The conventional order in which image data is collected and k-space is filled i.e., starting with the most negative phase encoding step and incrementing to the most positive step. It is usually denoted on DICOM images as SQ.

See also *centric k-space filling*.

SG

Abbreviation for the *SARGE* sequence used by Hitachi.

Shaded surface display

A common method of displaying images in 3D where light is artificially projected onto a *surface rendering* of the data to enhance the visualization.

See also *maximum intensity projection*.

Shielding

1. The process of reducing the extent or effects of a magnetic field. Shielding is used for both the main magnetic field and gradient fields and can be classified as either *active shielding* or *passive shielding*.
   See also *RF shielding*.
2. The screening effect of the surrounding electron clouds of atoms that reduce the magnetic field experienced by the nuclei.
   See also s*hielding constant*.

Shielding constant

A dimensionless quantity which characterizes the ability of the electron cloud of an atom to reduce the magnetic field experienced by the nucleus. The value increases with the number of electrons and varies from 10^{-6} to 10^{-2}.

See also *chemical shift*.

Shim

The end result of improving ("shimming") the *homogeneity* of the main magnetic field by adding small corrective fields. This is achieved by either *passive shimming* or *active shimming*.

Global shimming refers to the shim of the whole sensitive volume of the coil, whereas local shimming is applied to only a small volume of interest.

In MRS, the resulting homogeneity (or quality of the shim) is crucial for good resolution of spectral peaks. For typical peak widths see *FWHM* (Fig. 83).

See also *manual shim* and *auto shim*.

Shimadzu

Japanese based MRI vendor.

Shine through

Description of the appearance of an image when the desired weighting effect is dominated by a second effect e.g., at high *b-factor* values the diffusion decay should make the signal dark but may appear artificially bright in areas with long T_2 values (called T_2 shine through).

See also *exponential* ADC.

Shinnar-Le-Roux

The name of a specially shaped RF pulse with a sharp *slice profile*, which has superior definition compared to a conventional *sinc shaped* pulse.

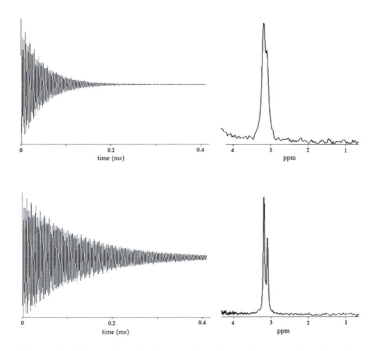

FIGURE 83 Examples of *shim* quality. In each case a time domain signal (FID) is shown on the left and its corresponding frequency spectrum shown on the right after applying a Fourier transformation. A poor shim (*top*) is characterized by a rapidly decaying FID and poorly resolved spectral peaks. Improving the shim (*bottom*) extends the FID and narrows the peak widths meaning the two peaks in this example can be distinguished

SHORT

Acronym of SHOrt Repetition Technique. A fast gradient-echo sequence that is similar to *FLASH*.

Short bore

The description applied to modern MRI systems which utilize the latest manufacturing technology in order to reduce the bore length. It is particularly used in conjunction with 3.0 T scanners, which can now be made with comparable lengths to that of some 1.5 T machines. The front-to-back dimension of a short bore 3.0 T scanner is around 1.7–1.9 m. The shortest 1.5 T system currently available is around 1.2 m in length (Fig. 84).

See also *long bore* and *wide bore*.

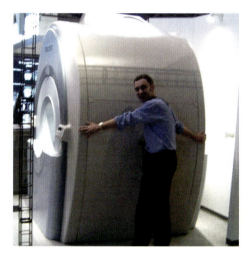

FIGURE 84   The author illustrates the *short bore* of this Toshiba system. Liney G. MRI in clinical practice. London: Springer; 2006, p. 23

Short tau inversion recovery

Commonly abbreviated to STIR. A specific *inversion recovery* sequence using a short *inversion time* (TI or denoted by the Greek letter tau, τ) as a method of *fat suppression*. At 1.5 T this value is around 180 ms. The signal is acquired as fat reaches the *null point* but water still has a non-zero magnetization. In the subsequent image only the water component contributes to the signal (Fig. 85).

See also *long tau inversion recovery*.

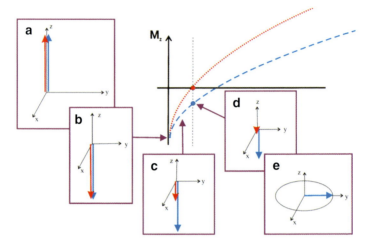

FIGURE 85 Diagram of the *short tau inversion recovery* (STIR) technique. (**a**, **b**) The water (*blue*) and fat (*red*) spins are first inverted with a 180° RF pulse. (**c**) The fat recovers quicker along the z-axis due to its shorter T_1 relaxation time. At the null point (**d**) the fat has a zero transverse component of magnetization (M_z). A 90° pulse is then applied (**e**) which turns the negative water peak into the transverse plane to be imaged

Shot factor

See *EPI Factor*.

Siemens (Healthcare)

German based **MRI** vendor offering a family of whole-body systems (called Magnetom) ranging from 0.35 to 3.0 T. Examples include the Trio (3.0 T), Avanto (1.5 T) and Espree (1.5 T *wide bore*).
www.medical.siemens.com

Signal

The coherent contribution to the image brightness.
See also *SNR* and *noise*.

Signal averaging

See *averaging*.

Signal difference to noise ratio

See *contrast-to-noise ratio*.

Signal-time curve

A commonly used method of analyzing *dynamic contrast enhancement* data. A region-of-interest is drawn in an image to produce a plot of signal intensity at each time point. This demonstrates the contrast uptake and wash-out characteristics from that region of tissue. The signal intensity is more usefully converted to percentage enhancement which is normalized by a pre-contrast value. Many measurements can be made from the curve including maximum enhancement, *enhancement rate* and *positive enhancement integral*. When this analysis is done on pixel-by-pixel basis a *parameter map* may be produced.

Signal-to-noise ratio

See *SNR*.

Silent word generation

A *paradigm* used in functional MRI in order to study language function in the brain. It typically requires the patient to complete a sentence or think of words beginning with a letter that is visually provided by a screen or video *goggles*. The patient is asked to not speak to reduce motion artifacts but also to distinguish *Broca's area* and *Wernicke's area*. This type of fMRI examination is a potential non-invasive alternative to the *Wada test*.

Silicon

A substance commonly found in breast implants which can be imaged with proton MRI. At 1.5 T it has a resonant frequency which is 100 Hz from fat (320 Hz from water).

Silicon-based oil is used in phantoms at high field owing to its lower *permittivity* which reduces the *dielectric effect*.

Silicon specific

The description of sequences that utilize both water and fat suppression in order to image the remaining silicone resonance from breast implant patients for investigation of rupturing etc.

Simultaneous excitation

A method of speeding up imaging time by acquiring two or more slices at once using *composite pulses*. The technique cannot be used where anatomy extends beyond the field-of-view in the phase direction. Examples include *POMP*, *dual slice* or *quadscan*.

Sinc shaped

A mathematical function described by:

$$\sin x \, / \, x$$

The sinc function is the *Fourier transformation* of a square wave function. Theoretically an infinitely long sinc shaped signal would provide a perfect *slice profile*. However, in practice with a finite pulse length, the actual profile becomes more rounded.

Sinerem

Commercial name for a *USPIO* type contrast agent used in liver imaging. It has been developed by AMAG Pharmaceuticals. It is generally referred to as Ferumoxtran and is also branded as *Combidex* with a previous research name of AMI-227.

See also *liver-specific contrast agents*.

Single dose

The quantity of contrast agent dose administered per unit of body weight. *Gd-DTPA* is licensed up to triple doses with a single dose equal to 0.1 mmol kg^{-1}.

Single-shot

Description of an ultra-fast imaging sequence (e.g., EPI) in which the entire k-space data is collected in one single repetition time (TR).

See also *EPI factor* and *multi-shot*.

Single voxel

MRS technique in which slice selection is performed in each orthogonal direction to localize the signal from the common intersection or *voxel*.

See also *MRSI*.

SINOP

Acronym for Simultaneous acquisition on IN and OPposite phase. A technique for producing images with fat and water signal both in phase and out of phase.

See also *chemical shift artifact* (*"of the second kind"*).

Skin depth

The finite penetration of radio-frequency into a conducting body. This has a consequence for the B_1 transmission, which at high field (>3.0 T) necessitates the use of increased *RF power*, which in turn accentuates the *SAR*. The RF skin depth is defined as:

$$\sqrt{2/\mu_o \mu_r \sigma \omega}$$

where μ_0 is the *permittivity* of free space, μ_r the relative permittivity of the sample, σ, conductivity, and ω, is the RF frequency. Skin depth also affects the *quality factor* of the RF coil.

See also *B_1 doming*.

Slab

The volume of tissue which is acquired in 3D imaging (see *imaging, 3D*). This is sometimes divided into partitions. Sometimes referred to as a chunk.

See also *Multi-slab*.

Slew rate

Specification of the imaging *gradient* which takes into account both the *rise time* and maximum amplitude. It is defined by:

Slew rate = amplitude / rise time

Units are in T m^{-1}s^{-1} and modern slew rates go up to 200 T m^{-1}s^{-1}.

Slice

The finite section of spins that are excited by the *slice selection* gradient.

See also *multi-slice*, *slice gap* and *slice profile*.

Slice gap

The space between consecutive imaging slices. Usually this is set to around 10% of the slice thickness to account for *cross excitation*. This should be increased to 20% for certain sequences (e.g., STIR). *Contiguous* slices are acquired with a zero gap. Slice gap is also known as slice spacing or slice interval.

Slice profile

The shape of the actual excited cross-section of spins. Ideally this should be rectangular and match the nominal slice thickness selected by the user. This would however, require an infinitely long *sinc shaped* pulse in the time domain. In practice, the pulse is truncated leading to a more rounded profile and causes *cross-excitation*. The actual slice thickness may be measured using a *profile phantom*.

Slice selection

The application of a finite bandwidth RF pulse in the presence of a linear gradient to excite a section of spins perpendicular to the direction of the gradient. The gradient has an initial *dephasing lobe* (negative amplitude) to ensure that spins are rephased at the center of the gradient (e.g., see Fig. 88). Slices can be acquired in either a *sequential* or *inter-leaved* manner (Fig. 86).

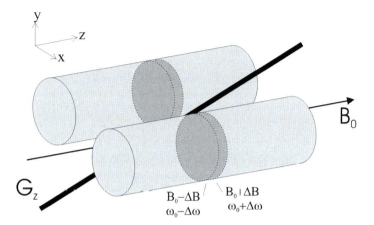

FIGURE 86 Illustration of *slice selection*. In this example an axial slice is acquired from two cylindrical samples. A gradient is applied along the z-direction (G_z) and this changes the field strength either side of the isocenter by $\pm\Delta B$. This changes the resonant frequency for a finite section of spins which can then be excited using an RF pulse with a bandwidth of $\pm\Delta\omega$. Liney G. MRI in clinical practice. London: Springer; 2006, p. 12

Slice thickness

The nominal width of the imaging slice set by the user and determined by the actual *slice profile*.

Slice warp

The deviation of the imaging slice from its intended perpen-dicular orientation with the slice selection gradient. It is inves-tigated using an appropriate test object, which consists of a series of angled rods, which run parallel to the slice direction.

Deviations from the actual rod separations reveal the degree of warping.

See also *quality assurance*.

Slice width

See *slice thickness*.

SLIP

Acronym for Spatial Labeling Inversion Pulse. A type of *arterial spin labeling* sequence from Toshiba.

SLR

Abbreviation for the *Shinnar-le-roux* pulse.

SMART

Acronym for Serial Motion Artifact Reduction Technique from Philips.

SMART Prep

GE's automatic initiation method of *bolus tracking* used in *contrast enhanced MRA*. The contrast agent is administered and when the baseline signal exceeds a certain threshold the scan is triggered. Similar techniques are known as *CARE bolus* (Siemens), BolusTrak (Philips), Visual Prep (Toshiba) and FLUTE (Hitachi).

SMASH

Acronym for the SiMultaneous Acquisition of Spatial Harmonics. A *parallel imaging* method for speeding up imaging time by replacing some of the phase encoding steps with linear combinations of receiver coils. Similar to *SENSE* but involves combining time domain signals with a knowledge of sensitivity profiles, prior to reconstruction i.e., it operates in k-space rather than in imaging space like SENSE.

References

Sodickson DK, Manning WJ. Simultaneous acquisition of spatial harmonics (SMASH): fast imaging with radiofrequency coil arrays. Magn Reson Med. 1997;38:591–603

SNR

Abbreviation of Signal-to-Noise Ratio. An important *quality assurance* parameter. It is equal to the *signal* from the imaging slice divided by the *noise* which is picked up from the entire *sensitive volume* of the receiver coil. SNR may be improved by using small anatomy-specific RF coils, large voxel sizes, signal *averaging* and operating at *high field* (see B_0). It becomes worse with increasing receiver bandwidth (see *variable bandwidth*).

SNR is measured in a *floodfill phantom*. There are several different methods for measuring SNR, and by applying appropriate factors these should be in agreement. The two main methods are:

1. Subtraction method: Two separate but otherwise identical images are acquired. SNR is taken to be equal to the mean signal in one image divided by the standard deviation (SD) in the subtracted images. A factor equal to 1.414 (= $\sqrt{2}$) is then applied.
2. Single image method: Mean signal in one image is divided by the SD of signal from a region in the background avoiding ghosts. A factor equal to 0.655 is applied (= $\sqrt{2 - \pi/2}$).

There are no ideal values for SNR and it is difficult to compare across systems unless *quality factor* and *filling factor* are accounted for. It remains a useful routine measure for monitoring deterioration in performance but is not very specific as to the cause of any problem.

SNR may be further normalized by dividing by the square root of the acquisition time to give the *efficiency* of a sequence.

SNR is also sometimes written as S/N (Fig. 87).

See also *NEX* and *contrast-to-noise ratio*.

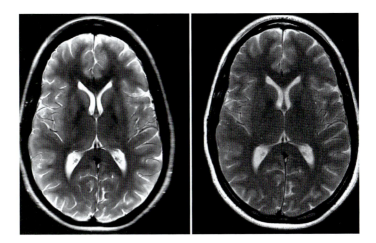

FIGURE 87 The image on the left has superior *SNR* compared to the image acquired at the same slice position on the right which looks much grainier. Liney G. MRI in clinical practice. London: Springer; 2006, p. 36

References

McRobbie DW. The absolute signal-to-noise ratio in MRI acceptance testing. Br J Radiol. 1996;69:1045–1048

Sodium

The MR visible isotope of sodium is ^{23}Na, and it has four energy states ($I = 3/2$). Sodium imaging is being increasingly used to detect elevated tissue sodium levels for example in myocardial infarction and cancer. It also increases in *HIFUS* allowing this treatment to be monitored.

MR properties of ^{23}Na:

Spin quantum number = 3/2
Sensitivity = 0.093
Natural abundance = 100.00%
Gyromagnetic ratio = 11.26 MHz T^{-1}.
See also *quantum number*.

References

Pabst T, Sandstede J, Beer M, Kenn W, Neubauer S, Hahn D. Sodium T_2^* relaxation times in human heart muscle. J Magn Reson Imaging. 2003;15:215 218

Sodium chloride

Added to water-based *phantoms* to adjust the conductivity to that of a typical patient. A concentration of around 0.33 g/100 mL is recommended.

See also *loading* and *saline*.

Soft tissue

Referring to the unique contrast capability of MRI permitting the imaging of internal soft-tissue organs. This is unlike CT which demonstrates bony anatomy well but has low soft-tissue contrast.

Solenoid

A very efficient RF coil design used to produce a magnetic field along the long axis of the coil. As such it is not particularly useful in conventional *horizontal bore* scanners but is used to good effect in vertical magnet designs. May be a single or multiple turn design (see Fig. 81).

Source data

The basic image data which is post-processed in some way to provide additional information (e.g., a *parameter map*). It is sometimes used interchangeably with the term *raw data*.

SPACE

Acronym for Sampling Perfection with Application optimized Contrasts using different flip angle Evolution. A Siemens 3D volume sequence with T_2 contrast. Equivalent to *CUBE* (GE) and *VISTA* (Philips).

SPAIR

Philips sequence similar to *SPIR* fat suppression but very insensitive to B_1 inhomogeneity. An acronym for Spectral Attenuated Inversion Recovery. Makes use of a delay to ensure that fat is in the correctly inverted position prior to imaging.

SPAMM

Acronym for SPAtial Modulation of Magnetization. Commonly used name given to *spin tagging* in cardiac imaging.

Spatial domain

The *Fourier transformation* of *time domain* data.

Spatial resolution

The nominal pixel size of the image determined (in-plane) by the FOV divided by the matrix size. Through-plane resolution is determined by *slice* thickness (in 2D imaging) or the *slab* thickness divided by a second phase encoding matrix in 3D imaging. The spatial resolution may be measured using a *resolution phantom*.

In MRS the resolution is equal to the volume of interest (VOI) divided by the phase encoding matrix.

See also *quality assurance*.

SPECIAL

Acronym for SPECtral Inversion At Lipids. A fat suppression method from GE utilizing a *spectral-spatial* pulse.

Specific absorption rate

See *SAR*

Spectral editing

Referring to a variety of methods, which take advantage of relaxation time or coupling differences in order to facilitate the identification of spectral peaks.

See also *TE averaging*.

Spectral resolution

The number of data points displayed in an MR *spectrum*. It refers specifically to the frequency range (known as the spectral or sweep width) of the data divided by the number of time domain points measured. Typically a ^{1}H spectrum may be acquired using a 2,500 Hz spectral width and 1,024 time domain points.

Spectral-spatial pulse

A type of spatially selective RF pulse that has a well-defined frequency bandwidth. Used primarily to not excite fat around the prostate and thereby improve spectral quality in this anatomy (see *PROSE*).

Spectroscopy

See *MRS*.

Spectroscopic imaging

See *MRSI*.

Spectrometer

Part of the scanner system, which is able to generate and detect discrete frequencies.

See also *pulse controller*.

Spectrum

A plot of signal amplitude against resonant frequency used to display and interpret *MRS* data.

SPEEDER

Name given to the image-based *parallel imaging* acquisition implemented by Toshiba systems.

SPGR

Abbreviation for SPoiled GRadient sequence.
  See also *FSPGR*.

SPIDER

Acronym for Steady-state Projection Imaging with Dynamic Echo-train Read-out. A multi-echo TrueFISP type sequence with spiral k-space acquisition that has been developed for *cardiac MRI*. Temporal resolution can be as little as 45 ms to enable real-time *cine* imaging.
  See also *spiral EPI*, and *k-space trajectory*.

Spin

The quantised (discrete) value of spin angular momentum possessed by a nucleus in a magnetic field. It is related to the spin *quantum number*. The term spin is often also used interchangeably for the magnetic *moment*.

Spin angular momentum

The momentum of an atomic particle due to the spinning on its axis. An electron also posses orbital angular momentum.

Spin density

See *proton density*.

Spin echo

The basic MRI pulse sequence using a 90° *excitation pulse* followed by a 180° *refocusing pulse* in order to recover T_2^*

decay and produce a signal echo which has decayed due to T_2 relaxation alone.

Signal in a spin-echo sequence is given by:

$$S \propto \left[1 - \exp(-TR/T_1)\right] \exp(-TE/T_2)$$

where *TE* and *TR* are the echo time and repetition time respectively.

Other types of echo produced in MRI are *gradient echo* and *stimulated echo* (Fig. 88).

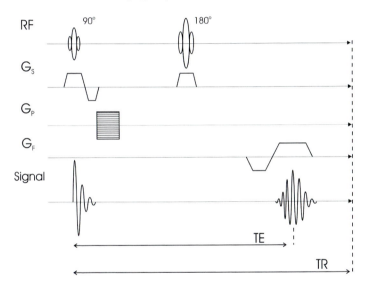

FIGURE 88 Pulse sequence diagram for the *spin echo* sequence. The 180° RF pulse is applied at TE/2 to produce an echo at time TE. G_S, G_P and G_F represent the gradients for the slice selection, phase encoding and frequency encoding respectively. The hatched lines of G_P indicate that this amplitude is varied incrementally for each TR. Liney G. MRI in clinical practice. London: Springer; 2006, p. 16

Spin-lattice relaxation

Synonym for T_1 relaxation.

Spin-spin coupling

See *J-coupling*.

Spin-spin relaxation

Synonym for T_2 relaxation.

Spin quantum number

See *quantum number*.

Spin states

The number of possible energy levels a *spin* can possess when placed in a magnetic field. A total of 2I+1 levels exist where I is the spin *quantum number*. The energy difference between these spin states increases linearly with magnetic field. For the *proton* (I = 1/2), there are two states referred to as *spin up* and *spin down*.

Spin tagging

Also known as myocardial tagging or *SPAMM*. A cardiac imaging method whereby rows and columns of spins are deliberately *saturated* in order to produce dark grid lines on the image. These are then used to visually monitor cardiac wall motion and thickness. A 1D equivalent method is also used. The darkness of the tags fades during the cardiac cycle due to T_1 recovery (Fig. 89).

Spin up/spin down

The two possible *spin states* of nuclei with I = 1/2 (for example a proton) when placed in a magnetic field. The lower energy

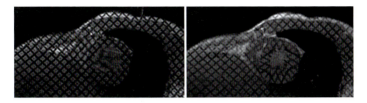

FIGURE 89 The use of *spin tagging* to superimpose grid lines across the image and aid in the visualization of cardiac wall motion. Note that the lines have slightly faded in the second image. Liney G. MRI in clinical practice. London: Springer; 2006, p. 105

spin-up state (sometimes denoted α), is where the spins are aligned with the field. The higher energy spin-down state (β) corresponds to anti-parallel alignment. At thermal equilibrium there is a slight majority of spins in the lower energy state causing an overall *net magnetization* in the direction of the field. Application of RF energy induces a transition between these two states (Fig. 90).

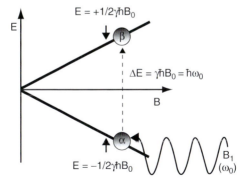

FIGURE 90 Energy level diagram for a proton in a magnetic field. The energy difference between the *spin up* (α) and *spin down* (β) states increases with field strength. Application of an RF pulse at resonant frequency causes a transition between these states

Spinor

The peculiar quantum physics property of the spin *wave function* where a 360° pulse is not equivalent to 0° but a 720° pulse is!

SPIO

Acronym for Super Paramagnetic Iron Oxide (pronounced "Es-pee-o"). A specific category of *contrast agents* which are derived from iron oxide coated particles of between 50 and 150 nm diameter. Their *relaxivity* is greater than gadolinium-based agents and is also a predominantly T_2 effect resulting in a signal decrease or negative enhancement effect.

See also *USPIO*.

SPIR

Acronym for SPectral saturation with *Inversion Recovery*. A method of fat suppression combining both chemical selective (*CHESS*) and *STIR* methods, implemented on Philips scanners.

See also *SPAIR*.

Spiral EPI

Type of EPI sequence whereby the gradients are played out in such a way so as to traverse k-space in a spiral direction.

See also *constant EPI*, *blipped EPI* and *k-space trajectory*.

Spline

A smoothly varying polynomial function that is used in the interpolation or smoothing of data. Its name comes from the device used by shipbuilders to draw smooth shapes. An example of its use is in the fitting of a spectral baseline in order to flatten the spectrum (see *rolling baseline*).

Splitting constant

A value which is related to the degree of interaction between coupled spins and determines the separation or splitting of these resonances in an MR *spectrum*.

See also *AB systems*.

Spoiling

The active destruction of transverse magnetization by applying appropriate gradients (gradient spoiling) or RF pulses (RF spoiling) at the end of the sequence. Used in rapid gradient echo techniques such as *FSPGR* and *FLASH* to avoid a steady-state build-up.

Spurious peaks

Artefactual peaks in an MR spectrum that are caused by a *susceptibility artifact*.

SQ

DICOM notation meaning image acquisition with SeQuential slices.

SS

Used as a prefix for sequences to indicate that they are acquired in a *Single-Shot*.

SSD

Abbreviation for *Shaded Surface Display*.

SSFP

Abbreviation for Steady State Free Precession. A sequence that is similar to *FIESTA* and *True FISP*.

SSP

Abbreviation for Sloped Slab Profile. The name of the variable flip angle technique from Hitachi used to reduce the saturation effects and increase sensitivity to *in-flow enhancement*.

See also *TONE*.

SSRF

Abbreviation for Spectral-Spatial RF. See *spectral-spatial pulse*.

Stability

1. The short-term consistency of the measured signal intensity during the scan. It is an important *quality assurance* measurement for *fMRI* indicating the flatness of the *baseline* signal. Ideally the percentage signal variation should change by no more than ±0.5% over several minutes. There should also be no discernible drift in the signal over the time course. It is measured by imaging a *floodfill phantom* and often a warm-up scan may be needed before the scanner performs in a stable fashion.

References

Weisskoff RM. Simple measurements of scanner stability for functional NMR imaging of activation in the brain. Magn Reson Med. 1996;36:643–645

2. The expected variation in the center frequency, quoted in ppm per hour, is referred to as the *field stability*.

STAGE

Acronym for Small Tip Angle Gradient Echo. A sequence that is similar to *FLASH*.

STAIR

Acronym for Solution and Tissue Attenuation Inversion Recovery. Pulse sequence, which uses two 180° inversion pulses each with a different *inversion time* (TI). Can be used in a similar way as a combined *STIR* and *FLAIR* sequence with TIs equal to 180 ms and 2 s in order to suppress fat and CSF in the brain and enable an improved visualization of gray matter.

References

Redpath TW, Smith FW. Use of a double inversion recovery pulse sequence to image selectively grey or white matter. Br J Radiol. 1994;67:1258–1263
    See also *inversion recovery*

Staircase artifact

The step-like appearance of 3D reformatted images that can occur when the slice thickness is too large to accurately represent the variation in the object contour.
    See also *reformat*.

Standing wave artifact

The variation in signal across an image observed at higher field strengths due to the reduced wavelength and *dielectric effect*.

See also *B_1 doming* and *wavelength*.

Static field limits

See *safety limits*.

Station

The patient table position during a *stepping table* acquisition. For example in *whole body screening* or *peripheral MRA* the imaging may be performed at three or more stations.

Statistical errors

Statistical errors may be classified into types. A type I error arises from using an inappropriately large *P-value* to assign significance to data, which results in a positive result only by chance. In statistical terms this equates to the null hypothesis being rejected falsely.

If the P-value is too small, a type II error results (the null hypothesis is accepted falsely), where real significance in the data is not detected (See *bonferroni correction*).

Type A errors can be classified as errors associated with repeat measurements and type B errors include all other errors.

References

Everitt BS. Medical statistics from A to Z. Cambridge: Cambridge University Press; 2003. ISBN: 0521532043

Steady state

The situation that exists after a train of rapid and closely spaced RF pulses are applied. If this is done so that $TR \ll T_2$ then the generated *FID* and *spin-echo* signals merge into a continuous signal of varying amplitude referred to as a steady-state free precession.

Steady-state sequence

Sequences, which maintain a transverse magnetization by using a TR shorter than T_2. True steady state sequences are sometimes called "coherent" whereas spoiled techniques, which actively dephase the transverse magnetization, can be called "incoherent."

See also *True FISP* and *GRASS*.

Steal effect

Term used to describe vascular supply which is taken from elsewhere due, for example, to arterio-venous malformation (AVM), and leading to possible functional impairment. This effect is also observed in tumors with poor vessel integrity.

STEAM

Acronym for STimulated Echo Acquisition Mode. Type of spectroscopy localisation sequence using three 90° RF pulses and slice selection in each orthogonal direction to excite the intersected volume or *voxel*. The sequence produces a *stimulated echo* with inherently less signal than *PRESS* but it has better voxel definition. *Crusher gradients* are used to remove unwanted signal echoes generated from the other pulse combinations.

References

Frahm J, Bruhn H, Gyngell ML, Merboldt KD, Hänicke W, Sauter R. Localized high-resolution proton NMR spectroscopy using stimulated echoes: initial applications to human brain in vivo. Magn Reson Med. 1989;9:79–93

Stejskal–Tanner

Eponymous sequence comprising of a bipolar gradient arrangement for use in diffusion weighted imaging (see *DWI*). More generally referred to as the *pulsed gradient spin-echo* scheme. Two gradients of opposite polarity are applied, meaning stationary tissue is equally dephased and rephased. Moving spins however, accrue a net phase loss and appear as a signal loss. By using large amplitude gradients the sequence is sensitized to diffusional motion.

See also *diffusion* and *b-factor*.

References

Stejskal EO, Tanner JE. Spin diffusion measurements: spin-echoes in the presence of a time-dependent field gradient. J Chem Phys. 1965;42:288–292

Stepping table

Technique where the patient is moved and imaged at several different positions (called a *station*) in order to obtain full whole-body coverage. It is used in peripheral angiography and *whole-body screening* studies. Also known as moving table and MobiTrak (Philips). The images in Figs. 24, 65, and 100 have been acquired with a three station stepping table acquisition.

See also *TIMCT*.

Stereotactic

The description of a device or procedure used for localisation in three dimensions. For example prior to surgical biopsy of brain tumors, an *MR visible* stereotactic frame attached to the skull may be imaged to accurately localize the tumor although frameless alternatives are now in use.

STERF

Acronym for Steady-state TEchnique with Refocused FID. A Shimadzu sequence similar to *SSFP*.

Stimulated echo

The type of echo produced from three or more RF pulses. The transverse magnetization created by the first pulse is "stored" in the longitudinal plane by the second pulse, and recalled by the third pulse. It is the basis of signal in the *STEAM* sequence.

In total five echoes are produced from the interaction of three pulses (one stimulated and four spin-echoes).

The signal of the stimulated echo is given by:

$$S \propto \frac{M_0}{2} \sin \alpha_1 \sin \alpha_2 \sin \alpha_3 \exp(-2t_a/T_2) \exp(-t_b/T_1)$$

where t_a and t_b are the times between the first and second RF pulses and $\alpha_1 \ldots \alpha_3$ are the flip angles of each pulse. For maximum amplitude, three 90° pulses are used (as in the case of STEAM).

STIR

Acronym for *Short Tau Inversion Recovery*.

Storage time

Another term for *mixing time*.

Stray field

Another term for *fringe field*.

Streak artifact

An imaging artifact that can occur in radial acquisitions. See *radial k-space*.

Stress-perfusion agent

A pharmaceutical that is administered to induce stress on the heart in the study of myocardial perfusion (see *cardiac MRI*). Agents include vasodilators (e.g., adenosine) and others, which enhance the contractility of the heart (e.g., dobutamine).

Stroke

Term used to describe the loss of brain function caused by the interruption of blood supply (see *ischemia*).

See also *DWI*.

Superconducting magnet

Type of magnet which consists of an air-cored electromagnet with windings constructed from material with zero electrical resistance below a *critical temperature*. Typically a *niobium-titanium* or niobium-tin alloy set in a copper core is used. This type of magnet accounts for 90% of MRI scanners in clinical use.

See also *permanent magnet* and *resistive magnet*.

Superior

Name used to describe the direction towards the patient's head and the opposite of *inferior*. It is at the top of a *sagittal* and *coronal* image (see Figs. 18 and 82).

Supine position

Imaging position with the patient lying on their back as opposed to the *prone position*.

Surface coil

The simplest RF coil design consisting of a loop of wire and used as a *receiver* only. The B_1 *profile* of the coil is poor, with an excellent signal-to-noise ratio (*SNR*) nearest to the coil plane, but which drops of quickly further away. This may be improved with *coil uniformity correction* methods.

The relationship between magnetic field and distance from the coil can be derived from the *Biot-Savart law*. Good SNR is obtained at distances equal to the radius of the coil.

Multiple surface coils can be combined to form an *array*.

Surface rendering

A 3D visualization technique where the outer or border pixels of a structure are segmented and displayed as a surface. This reduces the amount of data that has to be displayed and can speed up rotation of the images etc.

Surgical planning

The use of advanced MRI techniques (especially *fMRI*) to highlight sensitive functioning brain tissue so that this may be spared during surgery.

References

Golder W. Functional magnetic resonance imaging: Basics and applications in oncology. Onkologie. 2002;25(1):28–31

Survey scan

Another term for the initial *localiser* scan.

Susceptibility

Property of matter that determines how easily it becomes magnetized when placed in an external field. Usually denoted by the Greek letter chi (χ) and is related to the *magnetization* (M) produced in the material by the external field (H):

$$M = \chi H$$

Susceptibility is related to relative *permeability* μ_r by:

$$\chi = \mu_r - 1$$

Interactions between the field and the orbiting electrons within the material can either augment (*paramagnetic* and *ferromagnetic* material with $\chi > 0$) or disperse (*diamagnetic* material with $\chi < 0$) the external field.

Usually expressed as mass susceptibility per kilogram of material. Values for some common materials are as follows:

Water = −0.9
Sodium chloride = −0.64

Araldite = −0.63
Perspex = −0.5
Oxygen = +133.6
Units are $1 \times 10^{-8} \mathrm{kg}^{-1}$

http://www.kayelaby.npl.co.uk/general_physics/2_6/2_6_6.html

Susceptibility artifact

Characteristic signal voids and distortions present in the image due to differences in *susceptibility* between foreign objects and tissue or within tissue itself e.g., at air-tissue interfaces. These differences perturb the local B_0 field and cause a non-linearity in the gradient fields.

The phase loss as a result of this effect is given by:

$$\Delta \varphi = \gamma G_i \Delta r TE$$

where G_i is the local gradient caused by the susceptibility difference, Δr is the voxel size and TE the echo time. The effect is therefore worse with larger voxels and longer echo times. The artifact is also worse at high field.

Susceptibility artifacts also manifest as *spurious peaks* in MRS (Fig. 91).

Susceptibility weighted imaging

A method of imaging which relies on the *BOLD* effect and phase differences to produce contrast. It is particularly sensitive to venous blood with this specific application also known as BOLD venography. The technique uses an RF spoiled 3D gradient-echo sequence. Magnitude and phase data are acquired and the phase data is high-pass filtered to remove artifacts. These two images are then combined to enhance the weighting of the final image and often displayed as a *minimum intensity projection*. As well as veins it is useful for imaging hemorrhage and iron storage.

See also *spoiling* and *high pass filtering*.

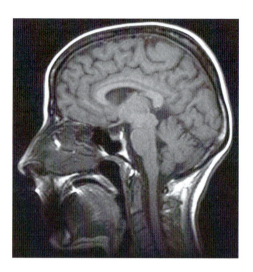

FIGURE 91 Dental work in this patient has caused a *susceptibility artifact* in this image. Liney G. MRI in clinical practice. London: Springer; 2006, p. 45

SVS

Abbreviation for Single Voxel Spectroscopy.

SWAN

GE's name for their *susceptibility weighted imaging* sequence.

Sweep width

See *spectral resolution*.

SWI

Abbreviation of *susceptibility weighted imaging* and also the name of the sequence used by Siemens.

Syrinx

A fluid filled cavity in the spinal cord, commonly seen in the cervical spine. *Gibb's artifact* present in the spine can often be mistaken for this.

T

T_1

The longitudinal or spin-lattice relaxation time. It is the time constant describing the recovery of the net magnetization (M_o) back to its re-alignment with B_0 following the removal of an *excitation pulse*. This return to equilibrium requires a loss of energy (to the surrounding lattice).

The magnetization in the longitudinal plane (z axis) is given by:

$$M_z = M_o \left(1 - \exp\left(-t / T_1\right)\right)$$

where M_0 is the net magnetization. At $t = 0$, $M_z = 0$ and as $t \rightarrow \infty$, $M_z = M_0$. T_1 is defined by the time taken for the M_z to recover to ~ 63% of M_0 (i.e., when $t = T_1$ the term above is $1 - e^{-1}$).

T_1 increases with field strength as $B_0^{1/3}$. It can be measured using an *inversion recovery* or *saturation recovery* sequence. Other specific sequences include *Look-Locker*.

Some example values of T_1 (at 1.5 T) are:

Water = 3,000 ms
CSF = 2,060 ms
Gray matter = 1,100 ms
Muscle = 1,075 ms
Breast tissue = 774 ± 183 ms[*]
White matter = 560 ms
Fat = 227 ± 42 ms[*]

*Authors own values

See also *relaxation* and *Bloembergen, Purcell and Pound equation*.

T$_1$-ρ

Pronounced "T$_1$ rho." This is the relaxation time used for describing the situation when the magnetization is locked in the *rotating frame*. It is dominated by T$_2$ processes and may be used as a contrast weighting.

References

Santyr GE, Fairbanks EJ, Kelcz F, Sorenson JA. Off-resonance spin locking for MR imaging. Magn Reson Med. 1994;32:43–51

T$_1$-weighted

Describing a sequence where signal contrast in the image is predominantly determined by differences in T$_1$ relaxation times. Also written in shorthand as T$_1$-W. A short echo time (*TE*) is used to minimize T$_2$-weighting together with a short repetition time (*TR*) (e.g., TR < 500 ms and TE < 50 ms). A T$_1$-weighted image is typically characterized by dark fluid signal due to the long T$_1$ relaxation time of water (Fig. 92).

T$_2$

The transverse or spin-spin relaxation time. This is the time constant that describes signal decay due to loss of phase due to spin-spin interactions. It is the part of the observed signal decay that cannot be recovered by a *refocusing pulse* (see *T$_2$**).

Unlike longitudinal relaxation times, T$_2$ remains relatively unchanged with increasing field strength. It can be measured using a *CPMG* or multi-echo FSE sequence.

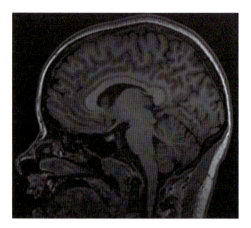

FIGURE 92 A sagittal T_1-*weighted* image of the brain using a spin-echo sequence with TE/TR = 9/380 ms. The long T_1 relaxation time of fluids makes the CSF appear hypointense

Some example values of T_2 (at 1.5 T) are:

Water = 3,000 s
Gray matter = 90 ms
White matter = 80 ms
Fat = 119 ± 5*
Breast tissue = 56 ± 12*
Muscle = 33 ms

* Authors own values

See also *relaxation*, *Bloembergen, Purcell and Pound equation* and *spin-echo*.

References

Poon CS, Henkelman RM. Practical T_2 quantitation for clinical applications. J Magn Reson Imaging. 1992;2:541–553

T_2^*

Pronounced "T-two-star." This is the effective or apparent transverse relaxation time. It is related to the dephasing of the net magnetization (M_o) following the removal of the *excitation pulse* B_1.

This causes a signal decay in the transverse plane (xy axis) that is referred to as the free induction decay (*FID*) and is given by:

$$M_{xy} = M_o \exp\left(-t / T_2 \,^*\right)$$

where M_0 is the net magnetization. At $t = 0$, $M_{xy} = M_0$ and as $t \to \infty$, $M_{xy} = 0$.

T_2^* is the time taken for the magnetization to decay to 37% of its initial value (i.e., when $t = T_2^*$ or the term above is equal to e^{-1}).

The term incorporates both the natural spin-spin T_2 decay component together with the effects caused by the inhomogeneities of the main magnetic field (often written as T_2'). The two effects combine such that:

$$1 / T_2 \,^* = 1 / T_2 + 1 / T_2'$$

It follows from above that T_2^* is always shorter than T_2. See also *spin-echo*.

T_2 map

A *parameter map* in which the pixel intensity represents the actual transverse relaxation time determined from at least two images of different echo times. Beginning to find use in cartilage imaging (Fig. 93) (see *cartigram*).

References

Nag D, Liney GP, Gillespie P, Sherman KP. Quantification of T_2 relaxation changes in articular cartilage with in situ mechanical loading of the knee. J Magn Reson Imaging. 2004:19;323–328

T_2 shine-through

See *shine through*.

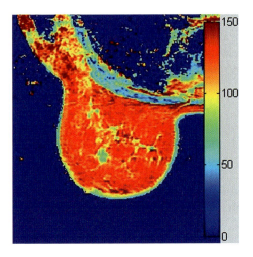

FIGURE 93 A T_2 *map* in a breast tumor patient produced from four FSE images with TEs ranging from 30 to 200 ms. The color scale gives T_2 values in millisecond

T_2-weighted

Description of an image in which the signal contrast is predominantly determined by differences in T_2 relaxation times. It is also seen written in shorthand as "T_2-W." A long repetition time (*TR*) is used to minimize T_1-weighting together with a long echo time (*TE*) (e.g., TR > 2,000 ms and TE > 100 ms). A T_2-weighted image is typically characterized by bright fluid signal due to the long T_2 relaxation time of water (Fig. 94).

T_2^*-weighted

An image that is essentially T_2-*weighted* albeit it is formed from a gradient echo so that the contrast is instead governed by T_2^*. These images will also be more prone to susceptibility effects and as such they are useful in detecting hemorrhage and also for *BOLD* imaging (Fig. 95).

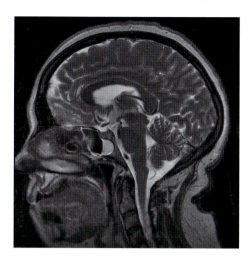

FIGURE 94 A sagittal *T$_2$-weighted* image of the brain using a fast spin-echo sequence with TE/TR = 100/4,000 ms. The long T$_2$ relaxation time of fluids makes the CSF appear hyperintense

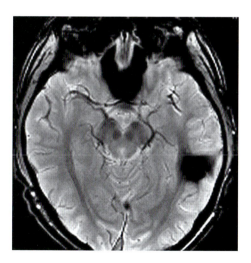

FIGURE 95 A *T$_2$*-weighted* gradient echo image demonstrates a hemorrhage due to the iron content which causes a signal decay. Liney G. MRI in clinical practice. London: Springer; 2006, p. 65

Tailored RF pulse

Term used to mean an RF pulse with a varying amplitude over time to create a optimal *slice-selection* pulse.

See also *sinc-shaped*.

Talairach space

The standard co-ordinate system used in the analysis of *fMRI* to enable different studies to be compared. The origin of this system is set to the line of the anterior and posterior commissure (or AC-PC line) and activation is then reported in x, y, z co-ordinates relative to this position.

References

Talairach J, Tournoux P. Co-planar stereotaxic atlas of the human brain. New York: Thieme; 1988

Tattoo

A permanent cosmetic or decorative tattoo may cause a transient *RF heating* effect or *susceptibility artifact* in the immediate vicinity due to iron-oxide particles in the pigment. As such a patient should be informed about the relatively small risk of a minor reaction and a cold flannel may also be applied onto the skin as a precaution.

Tau

Greek letter (τ) used to denote a time interval for example an inversion time (see *TI*) or *transit time*.

T_{del}

Shorthand used to denote the *temporal resolution* of a dynamic (multi-phase) scan. It is an abbreviation of the delay time.

TE

Abbreviation for echo time (or time to echo). The time at which the signal is recorded (see Fig. 88).

See also *refocusing pulse*.

TE averaging

A method used in MRS for eliminating the phase dependence of J-coupled resonances. Signal is collected at many different echo times so that the phase changes average out. This may be used to identify or remove *J-coupling* from the spectrum.

TEA-PRESS

Acronym for the *TE Averaging* version of the *PRESS* spectroscopy sequence.

Teleradiology

Term used to describe the viewing and reporting of medical images (often MRI) at a remote computer workstation.

See also *PACS*.

Temporal resolution

The time interval between successive acquisitions of the same slice or location in a *dynamic* scan. It is often abbreviated to T_{del}.

Typically a 3D volume may be acquired every 30 s, while 2D slices can be imaged every 1–2 s, using fast gradient echo methods. The temporal resolution is traded-off with higher spatial resolution or improved slice coverage. By combining advanced sequences and *parallel imaging* technology (e.g., *PRESTO* and *SENSE*) a whole brain scan can be imaged in as little as 1 s.

Tensor

Mathematically, a tensor of order n is a quantity requiring 3^n numbers to describe it. For example, a scalar is a zero order tensor (one number), a vector is first order (three components) and the diffusion tensor (see *DTI*) is second order (nine components).

Tesla

A relatively large unit of magnetic field compared to the *Gauss*, with 1 T equal to 10,000 Gauss. The highest magnetic fields currently produced in laboratories are around 30 T. Typical clinical MRI scanners range in field strength from 0.5 to 3.0 T.

Teslascan

The name of a liver specific contrast agent containing *manganese* (Mn-DPDP) developed by Amersham with a generic name of mangafodipir trisodium. It is a hepatobiliary agent, with a T_1 positive enhancement effect.

See also *liver-specific contrast agents*.

Test bolus

The injection of a small amount of contrast agent and timing its arrival at the site of interest in order to measure the *transit time*.

Test object

A device used to mimic the patient for *quality assurance* work.
See also *phantom*.

Tetramethylsilane

See *TMS*.

Textural analysis

A mathematical method by which the subjective interpretation of an MR image can be decomposed into a set of quantitative parameters which describe both the spatial variation and distribution of pixel values. The method has been applied to high resolution post-contrast images to describe enhancement patterns. It begins by first calculating a gray level co-occurrence matrix which determines how often intensity values occur in adjacent pixels. From this many parameters can be calculated often denoted by "f" numbers. Commonly used ones include angular second moment (or f1), contrast (f2), correlation (f3) and inverse difference moment (f5).

See also *morphological descriptors*.

References

Tourassi GD. Journey toward computer-aided diagnosis: Role of image texture analysis. Radiology. 1999;213:317–320

TG

Abbreviation for Transmitter Gain. System setting on GE scanners which adjusts the *transmitter* during the *pre-scan*.

Threshold

A limiting value which is used to instigate some event or process once it has been exceeded. Examples include; the minimum and maximum pixel intensity threshold used to define a range of pixels to be included in some image processing step; An ECG signal threshold used to trigger a gated sequence.

THRIVE

Abbreviation for T_1 High Resolution Isotropic Volume Examination. A Philips sequence, using a *SPIR* 3D T_1-weighted turbo spin-echo sequence combined with parallel imaging to obtain images with excellent spatial resolution and volume coverage in short *breath hold* examinations. Other equivalent sequences include *LAVA* (GE), *VIBE* (Siemens) and QUICK 3D (Toshiba).

TI

Abbreviation for either Time from Inversion or Time to Inspection but more commonly referred to as the inversion time in an *inversion recovery* sequence. It is equal to the time interval between the 180° inversion pulse and subsequent 90° pulse used to measure (or inspect) the signal in the transverse plane.

See also *null point* and *STIR*.

Time domain signal

The signal that is detected in the receiver coil prior to the *Fourier transformation* into the *spatial domain*.

Time-of-flight

See *TOF*.

Time-resolved MRA

Description of contrast-enhanced MR Angiography sequences whereby 3D volumes are acquired fast enough to permit the arterial and venous phases to be separately distinguished.

This negates the need for accurate *bolus timing* by acquiring data as quickly as possible. Names of some techniques include TRICKS, TRAQ, TRAK 4D and TWIST.

See also *4D scanning*.

Tip angle

Synonym for *flip angle*.

TIM

Acronym for Total Imaging Matrix. Siemens name for the ability of their systems to use multiple RF coils at once which can provide up to 200 cm imaging coverage for whole-body screening. Up to ten RF coils can be connected at any one time enabling the user to rapidly select the appropriate coil for imaging different anatomy.

TIMCT

Siemens utilization of their TIM technology along with a continuous moving table to enable constant imaging to be acquired in a similar manner to conventional CT scans. High reconstruction speed enables images to be displayed in real-time.

TIRM

Abbreviation for Turbo Inversion Recovery Measurement. A *long tau inversion recovery* sequence which is used to suppress fluid in a similar manner to *FLAIR*.

Titanium

Metallic element that has the highest strength-to-weight of any metal. Its non-ferromagnetism makes it a suitable material to be used for *MR compatible* equipment or devices (e.g., titanium biopsy needles).

TM

Abbreviation for the *mixing time*, in the *STEAM* spectroscopy pulse sequence.

TMS

1. Abbreviation for TetraMethylSilane. This is the reference compound used in both proton and carbon MRS (see *ppm*). It has 12 chemically identical protons which produce a single intense resonance far away from other peaks making it an ideal reference compound.
2. An abbreviation for *Transcranial Magnetic Stimulation*.

TNM staging

Common classification system used in cancer staging. A score is associated with the letters T, N and M, which stand for Tumor, Node and Metastases and used to indicate the extent and progression of the disease.

TOF

Abbreviation for Time-Of-Flight. A term that can be used to refer to any flow related phenomena used in MRA techniques, but nowadays used specifically to describe *in-flow enhancement* effects (Fig. 96).

References

Axel L. Blood flow effects in magnetic resonance imaging. AJR Am J Roentgenol. 1984;143:1167

TONE

Acronym for Tilted Optimized Non-saturated Excitation. A sequence using a variable flip angle across the imaging plane

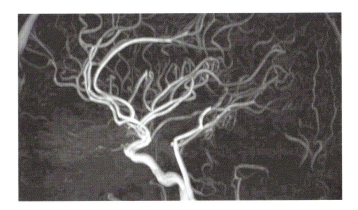

FIGURE 96 An example of a 3D *TOF* angiogram of the circle of Willis which has been displayed as a maximum intensity projection (MIP). Liney G. MRI in clinical practice. London: Springer; 2006, p. 112

in order to reduce the saturation effects and increase sensitivity to *in-flow enhancement*. Also known as *SSP* and *ramped RF pulses*.

Toshiba (Medical Systems)

MRI Vendor with current systems which include a 1.5 T (Vantage) with an extremely short *bore* length (see Fig. 84).
http://www.toshiba-medical.eu/en/Our-Product-Range/MRI
See also *Pianissimo*.

TR

Abbreviation for Time to Repetition, more commonly known as simply the repetition time. This is the time of each single unit of a pulse sequence i.e., the interval between successive excitation pulses. The TR is shown in Fig. 88.
See also *TE* and *flip angle*.

Trace

A rotationally invariant scalar measurement of the mean diffusivity derived from the diffusion tensor. It is sometimes wrongly expressed as the average apparent diffusion coefficient (ADC) in each imaging direction but is in fact given by:

$$\text{Trace} = \lambda_1 + \lambda_2 + \lambda_3 = 3 < D >$$

where λ_1, λ_2 and λ_3 are the *eigenvalues* from the diffusion tensor, and <D> is the mean diffusivity.

See also *DTI*.

TRAK, 4D

The name given to a *time resolved MRA* sequence from Philips.

Tractography

Term which describes the use of diffusion tensor imaging (see *DTI*) to identify fibers in tissue. Although it is being increasingly applied to other areas outside of the brain, the vast majority of work has concentrated on *white matter fibers*. Algorithms that seek out connectivity between diffusion directions (see *FACT*) are used to map out fiber trajectories in 3D. The technique can be useful in distinguishing tumor infiltration from displacement of tracts and the information can be used in surgery to spare functioning tissue.

Also known as fiber tracking.

References

Catani M, Howard RJ, Pajevic S, Jones DK. Virtual in vivo interactive dissection of white matter fasciculi in the human brain. Neuroimage. 2002;17:77–94

Transaxial

See *axial*.

TRANCE

Acronym for Philips' non-contrast enhanced MRA sequence. It stands for TRiggered Angiography No Contrast Enhancement. Siemens' version is called NATIVE, GE's version is InHance, Hitachi's is known as VASC and Toshiba have CIA and FBI.

Transceiver

An RF coil which is used as a combined *receiver* and *transmitter* for signal detection and excitation respectively. Examples include many head and body coils.

Transcranial magnetic stimulation

Abbreviated to TMS. This is a method whereby a hand-held figure-of-eight magnetic coil is placed on the scalp and used to stimulate or inhibit functional activation in the brain. It may be used in conjunction with fMRI to investigate brain function. *MR compatible* TMS coils exist which may be used on the patient whilst in the scanner.

References

Bohning DE, Shastri A, Nahas Z, Lorberbaum JP, et al. Echoplanar BOLD fMRI of brain activation induced by concurrent transcranial magnetic stimulation (TMS). Invest Radiol. 1998;33:336–340

Transit time

The time interval between the injection of contrast agent and its arrival at the site of interest. Also known as MTT (mean transmit

time) or τ. The value is very patient dependent (especially in the elderly) and it may be determined by first using a *test bolus*. This interval is then observed for the subsequent contrast enhancement study to ensure optimum timing of the sequence.

See also *contrast enhanced MRA*.

Transmitter

An RF coil that is only used to excite the MR signal.

See also *receiver*.

Transmitter reference voltage

A system setting on Siemens scanners which indicates the transmitter gain, which is adjusted during a *pre-scan*.

Transparency

Property of a fused data set which adjusts the degree to which either the underlying *primary image* or *secondary image* is visible. Sometimes referred to as the alpha value.

See also *overlay* and *fusion*.

Transverse

Another name for the *axial* (or transaxial) image orientation.

Transverse magnetization

See *net magnetization*.

Transverse plane

The name given to the plane which is perpendicular to the direction of the main magnetic field (B_0) and denoted the x-y plane by convention. This is where the net magnetization is detected by the RF coil and T_2 and T_2* relaxation effects occur in this plane leading to their alternative name of transverse decay.

See also *longitudinal plane.*

Trapezoid

The actual shape of the gradient amplitude produced by a gradient coil owing to the finite *rise time* (as opposed to the perfect rectangular shape).

TRAPS

Acronym for TRAnsitions between PSeudo-steady state. An imaging sequence designed to reduced *SAR* at high fields.

See also *hyperechoes.*

TRAQ

Acronym from Time Resolved AcQuisition. A *time-resolved MRA* sequence from Hitachi.

Travel SAT

See *moving saturation pulse.*

TRICKS

Acronym for Time Resolved Imaging of Contrast KineticS. A GE *key-hole imaging* sequence which permits high temporal and spatial resolution of contrasted enhanced MRA. Equivalent sequences include TWIST from Siemens, 4D TRAK from Philips, Freeze Frame from Toshiba and TRAQ from Hitachi.

See also *time-resolved MRA.*

Triggering

A term used interchangeably with the word *gating* to describe the synchronization of the imaging sequence with either cardiac or respiratory motion. It may also be used to refer to the initiation of some sequence, for example in *bolus tracking*.

Trigger window

The time interval between data acquisition and the detection of the next R-wave in cardiac gating. It is sometimes expressed as a percentage of the *RR interval* and also known as the *arrhythmia rejection* window.

TRSG

Acronym for Time Reversed *SARGE*. Name of a sequence from Hitachi that is similar to *PSIF*.

True FISP

A type of FISP sequence in which the transverse magnetization is preserved at the end of the *TR*. This utilizes *rewinding gradients* in all three directions rather than just the phase direction as in a normal *FISP* sequence. This requires high performance gradients and good shimming. Problems with the sequence lead to *banding artifacts*.

See also *ROAST* and *CISS*.

Truncation artifact

Synonym for ringing or *Gibb's artifact*. It occurs as a result of the finite number of samples that can be measured which equates to a truncation or under-representation of the Fourier series (see *Fourier transformation*).

The MR signal, may also be said to have been truncated if the receiver is not adjusted properly to accommodate high values, although this is more correctly referred to as data clipping (see *over-ranging*).

TSE

Abbreviation for Turbo Spin Echo. The Siemens version of the *FSE* sequence.

t-Test

Also known as students t-test. A common statistical test used to compare the differences between the mean values of sample data. It is the simplest test used in fMRI and involves comparing the mean "ON" values to the mean "OFF" values. The test result is assigned some degree of significance with an associated *P-value*.

See also *Z-score* and *bonferroni correction*.

Tumor

A solid growth, which may be either benign or malignant (cancer). The tumor can arise from local cells (primary) or from other sites (metastatic). Common brain tumors include gliomas and astrocytomas (malignant) and meningiomas (benign). MRI is extremely useful in imaging cancer due to its excellent soft-tissue contrast.

See also *TNM staging*.

Tunnel

Referring to the patient *bore* of a conventional *closed scanner* design.

Turbo dark fluid

The name of a *long tau inversion recovery* sequence which works in a similar manner to *FLAIR*.

Turbo factor

Synonym for the *echo train length* in a TSE sequence.

Turbo FLASH

Siemens ultra fast gradient echo sequence equivalent to *FSPGR* (GE) and Turbo Field Echo (Philips).
    See also *FLASH*.

Twin gradients

The design of two separate gradient coils operating over different linear extents and amplitudes. When a high gradient performance is required imaging can be switched to the smaller-sized gradient coil to prevent *peripheral nerve stimulation*.

TWIST

A *time-resolved MRA* sequence from Siemens.

Two (three)-compartment model

Physiological model used to interpret *dynamic contrast enhancement* data. The model incorporates compartments for blood, tumor and (additionally) extracellular-space. The data shown in Fig. 67 has been fitted using a two-compartment model.
    See also *pharmacokinetic modeling*.

References

Tofts PS, Brix G, et al. Estimating kinetic parameters from dynamic contrast-enhanced T_1-weighted MRI of a diffusible tracer: standardized quantities and symbols. J Magn Reson Imaging. 1999;10:223–232

Two-dimensional spectroscopy

See *NMR*.

Type I, II, III

Three stage classification of a *dynamic contrast enhancement* time course used in the diagnosis of tumors (especially breast). A Type I curve is described as having a gradual uptake over the time course and is generally linked to benign tumors. Type II describes a higher amplitude uptake that reaches a plateau and is typical of many malignant but also some benign tumors. Type III demonstrates rapid wash-in and wash-out rates and represents most malignant tumors and some fibroadenomas (Fig. 97).

   See also *BI-RADS*.

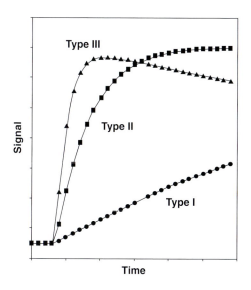

FIGURE 97 Simulated signal-time data representing each of the *Type I, II, III* dynamic contrast enhancement curves

U

Ultra-fast imaging

A phrase used to cover a whole host of rapid sequences and techniques that have been developed principally to alleviate problems from patient motion. They can be divided roughly into three categories: single shot techniques (e.g., *EPI*), partial k-space acquisition (e.g., *HASTE*) and those that use the additional hardware and post-processing required for *parallel imaging*.

Ultra-short TE

A description of sequences that use very short echo times (of the order of 0.08 ms) in order to visualize tissues with short T_2 components e.g., bone, ligaments and tendons.

Uniformity

A measure of how homogenous the signal intensity is within the image. The most significant contribution to this is the B_1 *profile* of the *RF coil* (see B_1 *inhomgeneity*).

Uniformity is measured in a *floodfill phantom* by one of two methods:

1. Line profile method: A pixel intensity profile is taken across the image (usually an average of multiple lines to improve signal-to-noise) to demonstrate the uniformity visually. It is advisable to avoid the edges if the phantom is a sphere rather than a cylinder. The fractional uniformity can be measured as the number of pixels that are within ±10% of the modal value found from a small central region-of-interest (ROI).
2. ROI method: A region is drawn at the center of the image and the percentage uniformity is defined as:

$$\%U = 100 \times \left(1 - \frac{\sigma}{S}\right)$$

where σ and S are the standard deviation and mean pixel intensity values from the region. Perfect uniformity will give a value of 100%.

See also *quality assurance*.

URGE

Acronym for Ultra-Rapid Gradient Echo. An imaging sequence which is a hybrid of the *burst imaging* technique and the *FLASH* sequence.

USPIO

Abbreviation for Ultrasmall Super Paramagnetic Iron Oxide. Note that the letter P in the abbreviation is sometimes defined as "Particulate."

A specific type of *contrast agent* comprising of iron oxide particles in a colloidal suspension. The "ultrasmall" applies to particles of <50 nm in diameter in comparison to *SPIO* agents and they may be further classified as *nanoparticles*. They are used extensively in imaging of the liver, nodal chains etc. Commerical examples include Sinerem, Resovist and Endorem.

The *relaxivity* of the iron oxide particles may be further increased by doping them with *manganese* to produce an ultrasensitive agent (increasing the relaxivity from around 150 to 358 mM^{-1}s^{-1}).

UTE

Abbreviation for *Ultra-short TE*.

V

Vacuum bore

An evacuated layer in between the gradient coils and patient bore used to reduce *acoustic noise* caused by the vibrating gradients. Approximately 20 dB reduction in noise can be achieved with this method.

See also *Pianissimo*.

Variable bandwidth

An imaging option which allows the *receiver* bandwidth (BW) to be manually adjusted. This effects the frequency difference between pixels and as such influences the *chemical shift artifact*. Some systems refer to this as optimized or matched bandwidth. Alternative names include *bandwidth per pixel* or water-fat shift.

Signal-to-noise ratio (see *SNR*) is also affected by changes in BW as it is inversely proportional to √BW (Fig. 98).

See also *bandwidth*.

Variable flip angle

See *ramped RF pulses*.

VASC

Acronym for Veins and Arteries Sans Contrast. Name of the non contrast enhanced sequence from Hitachi for renal and peripheral MRA. Similar sequences include TRANCE (Philips), InHance (GE), NATIVE (Siemens) and FBI/CIA (Toshiba).

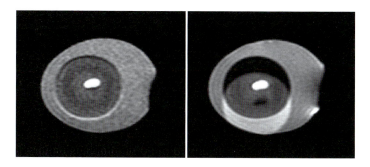

FIGURE 98 Images of an egg illustrate how adjusting the *variable bandwidth* affects an image. The bandwidth has been set to (*left*) 64 kHz and (*right*) 8 kHz. The reduction in bandwidth improves SNR but also generates a much larger chemical shift artifact. Liney G. MRI in clinical practice. London: Springer; 2006, p. 46

Vasovist

Commercial name of a *blood pool agent* (from Epix, Mallinckrodt, Bayer Schering Pharma). Its generic name is Gadofosveset trisodium and it has also been referred to as MS-325. The agent works by binding to blood protein albumin which extends its vascular half-life. The T_1 *relaxivity* is approximately ten times that of *Gd-DTPA*.

Vectorcardiogram

A spatial representation of the magnitude and direction of the cardiac signal abbreviated to VCG. This permits a near 100% triggering accuracy compared to normal *ECG gating* by using a more reliable R-peak detection algorithm.

See also *PQRST wave*.

Velocity encoding

The method of sensitizing the imaging sequence to flow by using *bipolar* gradients.

See also *phase contrast* and *VENC*.

VEMP

Acronym for Variable Echo MultiPlanar. A multiple spin-echo sequence from GE, which unlike *MEMP* may use variable echo spacing between the echoes.

VenBOLD

The name of a *susceptibility weighted imaging* sequence from Philips.

VENC

Acronym for Velocity ENCoding. This is the system parameter that adjusts the strength of the *bipolar* gradient in a *velocity encoding* sequence. Its value is the maximum velocity, which will be discriminated by the flow sensitive sequence. If this value is set too low then flow is not visible and vascular plaques will be overestimated. Typical blood velocities are 500 cm s^{-1} on exiting the heart, 80–175 cm s^{-1} in other arteries and down to 20 cm s^{-1} in the veins.

Vent

The airway between the top of scanner and the ceiling through which cryogen gases may exit safely during a *quench*. Also termed a *quench pipe* and examples of which can be seen in Fig. 48.

Venetian blind artifact

An artifact often seen in TOF angiography (see *in-flow enhancement*). It is due to discontinuities in adjacent slices or volumes, due to motion or saturation differences.

See also *CHARM*.

Venography

Imaging of veins with *susceptibility weighted imaging*.

Ventilation agent

A gas which is used as a contrast agent in MRI ventilation imaging. Examples include hyperpolarized gases (xenon, helium), 100% oxygen and less commonly gadolinium-based aerosols.
    See also *hyperpolarized gas imaging*.

Ventilation imaging

Imaging of the lung parenchyma following the inhalation of an appropriate *ventilation agent*.
    See also *hyperpolarized gas imaging* and *lung MRI*.

VERSE

Acronym for VariablE Rate Selective Excitation. A GE method of reducing SAR by up to 60%. It also offers improvements in image quality and T_2 contrast.

Vertical bore

The design of the scanner where the direction of the main magnetic field is perpendicular to the axis of the patient. The type of magnet orientation usually found in an *open scanner*.
    See also *horizontal bore*.

Vertigo

The sensation of dizziness or loss of balance sometimes experienced in fields of 4.0 T and above. This is due to rapid head movements inside the scanner bore but similar effects have been anecdotally reported near to the bore entrance of short bore lower field systems. Vertigo is often confused with the fear of heights (called acrophobia) but the sensation brought on by this is more correctly termed "height vertigo."

See also *bioeffects*.

VFL

Abbreviation for Variable FLip angle. This term refers to sequences using a *reduced flip angle* in order to reduce *SAR* at high field.

See also *hyperechoes* and *TRAPS*.

Viability imaging

See *delayed contrast enhancement*.

VIBE

Acronym for Volume Interpolated Body Examination. A Siemens *breath hold* sequence used in the abdomen. It utilizes *zero-filling* at the edges of the volume. Equivalent sequences include *LAVA* and *THRIVE*.

VIBRANT

Acronym for Volume Imaging for BReast AssessmeNT. A GE dedicated breast imaging sequence designed to permit *shim* in each separate well of the breast coil. This permits high definition bilateral breast imaging in one scan. Variants include VIBRANT-XV with accelerated imaging and VIBRANT-Flex with a 2-point *DIXON* sequence. Equivalent sequences are VIEWS (Siemens), BLISS (Philips) and RADIANCE (Toshiba).

VIE

Abbreviation for Virtual Intravascular (or Intraluminal) Endoscopy.

See also *virtual endoscopy*.

VIEWS

Siemens bilateral breast imaging sequence.

See also *VIBRANT*.

VIPR

Acronym for Vastly undersampled Isotropic Projection Reconstruction (pronounced "viper"). A method which uses a spherical k-space trajectory in order to obtain 3D image data with isotropic spatial resolution very quickly for use in dynamic *contrast-enhanced MRA*.

Virchow-Robin spaces

The small perivascular spaces in white matter, which become visible at very high field (around 5.0 T and above).

Virtual endoscopy

Technique of post-processing 3D MRI data in such a way as to simulate the "fly through" visualization of real endoscopy. Also referred to as Virtual Intraluminal Endoscopy (or VIE).

VISTA

Pulse sequence acronym for Volume ISotropic T_2-weighted Acquisition. A high spatial resolution sequence from Philips that can also be used with FLAIR. Equivalent to GE's *CUBE* and Siemens *SPACE* sequences.

Visual Prep

Toshiba's name for their version of *bolus tracking*.

VINNIE

Acronym for Velocity ImagiNg iN cInE mode. The use of dynamically acquired *phase-contrast* images to image blood flow.

VOI

Abbreviation of Volume-Of-Interest. A region-of-interest (ROI) in three dimensions. Often used to refer to the local-ized volume in MR spectroscopy.

Voxel

Word derived from "volume element" implying the 3D equivalent of the term *pixel*. It is almost exclusively used to describe the smallest volume of MRS data. It can also be used generally to refer to pixels in an image when the slice thick-ness is also considered.

Voxel bleeding

The unavoidable side-effect, due to the encoding used in MRI, whereby signal from any given voxel is displaced into other voxels in the rest of the image. Voxel bleed also means that the actual resolution is always worse than the nominal voxel size. It may be reduced by using spatial *apodisation* (e.g., a *Hanning filter* or *Fermi filter*), but this also leads to an increase in voxel size. The degree of voxel bleed increases as the number of phase encoding steps decreases therefore the effect is usually negligible for imaging but often severe for *MRSI*.

See also *point spread function*.

Voxel shifting

The technique of retrospective adjustment of the voxel position during the post-processing of *MRSI* data.

V/Q

Short-hand meaning ventilation and perfusion.
See also *ventilation imaging.*

VSS

Abbreviation for Very Selective Saturation. GE name for *saturation pulses* with well-defined spatial extent. Used primarily to improve the sharpness of voxel edges in MRS, and sometimes to eliminate unwanted signal from areas like frontal sinuses (*susceptibility artifact*) and scalp (too much fat).

Wada test

A highly invasive procedure in which a barbiturate is injected into one or other of the carotid arteries to anesthetise one side of the brain. The patient then undergoes tests to try to lateralise language function prior to surgery. Functional MRI (*fMRI*) is being increasingly used to replace this test by using an appropriate *paradigm* for example *silent word generation*.

Walking SAT

See *moving saturation pulse*.

Warning sign

Mandatory notification sign used to indicate the proximity of the high magnetic field of a scanner.

Wash in (out)

The rate at which *contrast agents* are taken up (or removed) by a tissue. Both are important in the differentiation of benign and malignant tumors.

See also *angiogenesis* and *pharmacokinetic modeling*.

Water

The principal source, along with fat, of proton signal in the human body. It is vastly more concentrated than other metabolites, requiring *water suppression* in MRS in order to visualize these other signals. It has a characteristic resonance of 4.7 ppm.

Water-fat shift

The name for the system parameter on Philips scanners which adjusts the *variable bandwidth*.

Water fraction

The relative amount of water signal in relation to the fat signal which may be measured using MRS or water and fat only imaging techniques (e.g., *IDEAL*, *DIXON*).

See also *fat fraction*.

Water-only image

An image created from the signal from the water resonance only and not the combined water and fat signal as in a routine image sequence. This is usually produced from the summation of an *in-phase image* and *out-of-phase image* in sequences such as *DIXON* (see Fig. 29).

See also *chemical shift* (*"of the second kind"*) and *fat-water in-phase*.

Water reference

The acquisition of MRS without *water suppression* to enable the water resonance to be used in some manner. Typically, the water signal is used to provide *absolute peak area quantification* or B_0 correction.

Water suppression

The removal of the water signal using a *CHESS* type pulse centered on the main proton frequency. It is used mainly in proton MRS to reduce the dominant water peak from the spectrum permitting the visualization of metabolites present at extremely low concentrations. The remaining water peak following suppression is referred to as the *residual water* (Fig. 99).

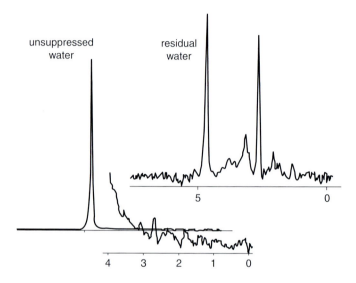

FIGURE 99 A proton spectrum from the prostate before and after *water suppression*. Water dominates the other resonant frequency signals (as shown by the magnified *inset*). After reducing the water signal 400-fold the lower concentration metabolites become visible. The residual water signal can be used as a chemical shift reference

WATS

Acronym for WATer Selection. A Philips sequence that excites water-only as a method of fat suppression.

Watt

The unit of power or rate of energy conversion (W) defined as $1 \, J \, s^{-1}$. Specific absorption rate (see *SAR*) is measured in $W \, kg^{-1}$.

Wavelength

The distance of one complete cycle of a waveform i.e., from one peak to the next. In MRI the wavelength of RF used is related to the magnetic field strength and dielectric constant or *permittivity* (ε) of the medium being imaged by:

$$\lambda = \frac{1}{\sqrt{\varepsilon}B_0}$$

At 3.0 T the wavelength in soft-tissue is approximately 26 cm which becomes comparable to the diameter of the patient and causes B_1 *doming*. In phantoms this effect can be remedied by using oil (low dielectric constant) instead of water as the filling solution.

See also *frequency*, *dielectric effect* and *dielectric pad*.

Wave guides

Holes in the scan room wall made of tubes with a frequency specific length-to-diameter ratio. These prevent RF entering the scan room but allow equipment to be passed into the room (e.g., patient monitoring equipments leads).

Wave function

Quantum mechanical description of a spin in the presence of a magnetic field, acknowledging that it exists as a linear combination of quantised states. It is usually given the Greek letter psi (Ψ).

See also *quantum number*.

WEFT

Acronym for Water Elimination Fourier Transform. A method of suppressing water used in MRS. It works by performing an *inversion recovery* pulse on the water peak followed by excitation of the remaining metabolites as the water reaches its *null point*.

Weighting

Term describing the degree and type of image contrast in MRI. For example an image can be described as being "heavily T_2-*weighted*" meaning its appearance is predominantly governed by differences in T_2 relaxation times.

See also T_1-*weighted*.

Weinmann data

Published measurements of the blood plasma concentration of Gd-DTPA over time. This can be used in *pharmacokinetic modeling* of contrast enhanced data.

References

Weinmann HJ, Laniado M, Mutzel W. Pharmacokinetics of Gd-DTPA/dimeglumine after intravenous injection into healthy volunteers. Physiol Chem Phys Med NMR. 1984;16:167–172

Wernicke's area

Part of the temporal lobe of the brain responsible for the interpretation of sound (the auditory association area).

See also *Broca's area*.

Whisper sequence

Term used generally to describe imaging sequences with very low gradient noise. Whisper gradients are specially designed gradient coils to reduce the *acoustic noise*.

White blood

Phrase referring to any MR Angiographic technique in which blood (flowing spins) appears brighter than stationary tissue.
See also *in-flow enhancement*.

White matter fibers

Bundles of neurons in the white matter that transmit nerve impulses from one part of the brain to another. The neurons are myelinated (insulated with fatty tissue) which makes them appear white. The fibers can be visualized with MRI owing to the preferred diffusion of water along their trajectories (see *DTI*). Three types of fibers exist: *association fibers*, *commissural fibers* and *projection fibers*.

Whole-body

1. Term used to describe the majority of clinical MRI systems that are capable of scanning all parts of anatomy. This distinguishes them from some systems (especially at higher fields) which, although physically covering the whole patient can only image with the RF head coil ("head only").
2. The name of the lower amplitude gradient set that extends over full coverage in systems with *twin gradients*.

Whole-body screening

Refers to an MRI examination in which a complete head-to-foot investigation is performed (for example to examine metastatic spread), using the body coil or separately selectable coil elements. These scans utilize a *stepping table* technique (Fig. 100).
See also *DWIBS*.

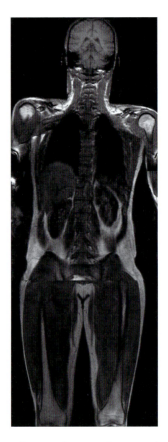

FIGURE 100 Images from a three-station stepping table technique have been pasted together to provide a *whole-body screening* study

Wide bore

Referring to closed MRI systems that have a patient *bore* around 70 cm or greater in width. This extra space offers some of the advantages of an *open scanner* with similar imaging quality to a tunnel system, although with slightly worse B_0 *inhomogeneity* than equivalent narrower systems of the same length.

See also *short bore*.

Width

1. The range of pixel values used to display the image.
   See also *windowing*.
2. The nominal slice thickness.
   See also *slice profile*.

Windowing

The manipulation of the pixel values displayed in an image to best show the contrast and detail (see Fig. 47). Although no change is made to the image data, only a user-specified range is displayed on screen. Usually both the window width and level are specified. Window width is the range of pixel intensities that are displayed as screen brightness and is related to image contrast. Window level is the mid-point of the window width and determines brightness. Most scanners automatically adjust the window settings following image acquisition but this may require fine-tuning by the operator, especially when viewing the background signal to evaluate ghosting or noise.

X

Xenon

The MR visible isotope of xenon is [129]Xe which may be used in *hyperpolarized gas imaging*. It has an advantage over helium in that it dissolves in the blood with a 200 ppm change in chemical shift between the liquid and gas phase meaning it can be studied with *MRSI*.

References

Albert MS, Cates GD, Driehuys B, et al. Biological magnetic resonance imaging using hyperpolarized [129]Xe. Nature. 1994;470:199–201.

x-direction

One of the directions in the transverse plane which is perpendicular to the main magnetic field *orientation*, and conventionally chosen as left to right (see Fig. 64).

Y

y-direction

One of the directions in the transverse plane which is perpendicular to the main magnetic field *orientation*, and conventionally chosen as the anterior-posterior direction (see Fig. 64).

Z

Z2 or Z4

Notation used to indicate an interpolation of spatial resolution in the slice direction by either a factor of 2 or 4.

See also *ZIP*.

z-direction

The head-to-foot imaging direction, or the *orientation* parallel to the main magnetic field and called the longitudinal plane (see Fig. 64).

Z-score

A standard score used in statistics to indicate how many standard deviations a measure is from the mean value. The letter Z refers to a normal population or "Z-distribution." The score is normalized by subtracting the mean value from the measurement and dividing by the standard deviation. When population values of mean and standard deviation are not known a *t-test* is used.

Zebra artifact

Alternative name for the appearance of *Moire fringes.*

Zeeman levels

The quantised energy states which arise in nuclei (or electrons) when they are placed in a magnetic field (see Fig. 90).

See also *quantum number.*

Zero filling

A method of appending zeros at the end, middle or beginning of the time domain signal to improve the *spectral resolution* in *MRS*. For example a spectrum acquired with 1,024 data points may be zero-filled to 2,048 points. Zero-filling in the time domain has the same effect as interpolation in the frequency domain.

Zeugmatography

Term derived from the Greek word Zeugma (meaning joining together). First used by Lauterbur to describe the combination of a static and RF magnetic field in order to produce MRI.

ZIP

Acronym for Zerofill InterPolation. A post-processing method used to artificially obtain images at a higher matrix size e.g., 1,024 from 512 data. This improves the apparent spatial resolution but at the expense of increased *ringing* artifacts.

Zipper artifact

Alternative name for an *RF artifact*.

Zoom gradients

See *twin gradients*.

Zoom imaging

Philips technique for *ultra-fast imaging* in real-time. It utilizes a very small field-of-view and reduced k-space to rapidly image at high resolution. The 90° and 180° pulses are applied perpendicular to each other to overcome phase wrap.